# *Advances in Neurotraumatology*

*Published under the Auspices of the Neurotraumatology Committee of the World Federation of Neurosurgical Societies*

*Editor-in-Chief: R. P. Vigouroux*

*Volume 2*

# *Thoracic and Lumbar Spine and Spinal Cord Injuries*

*Managing Editor: Ph. Harris*



Springer-Verlag Wien GmbH

Professor Robert P. Vigouroux
Clinique Neuro-chirurgicale, C.H.U. Timone, Marseille, France

Phillip Harris, F.R.C.S.E., F.R.C.P.E., F.R.C.S. (Glas.), F.R.S.E.,
Consultant Neurosurgeon, Department Surgical Neurology,
Western General Hospital, Edinburgh, Scotland



Originally published by Springer-Verlag Wien New York in 1987

With 64 Figures

ISSN 0178-3696

ISBN 978-3-7091-4145-8 ISBN 978-3-7091-4143-4 (eBook)
DOI 10.1007/978-3-7091-4143-4

# Foreword

Owing to their frequency and possible consequences and considering the fact they frequently affect young people, traumatic lesions of the thoraco-lumbar spine represent a special point of interest within the field of Neurotraumatology. Traffic accidents are the commonest cause, which accounts for the high peak of occurrence between 15 and 24 years of age. It is also worth noting that according to published series nearly 50% of the cases affect the thoraco-lumbar junction.

From an anatomical point of view, we must note the severity of thoracic spinal cord lesions especially of the thoraco-lumbar junction and of the lumbar region and be able to associate injuries of the conus medullaris and of the cauda equina where there is a possibility of neurological recovery.

Clinical evaluation is not always easy, but remains the basis for diagnosis and prognosis. The neurological classification proposed by FRANKEL *et al.* in 1969 and used at STOKE MANDEVILLE Hospital seems to retain its value. A more sophisticated study of medullary evoked potentials, as described by TSUBOKAWA can allow a more precise localisation and appreciation of the extent of the lesion as well as a better evaluation of the prognosis and of the evaluation of treatment in the acute phase.

The neuro-radiological study should include standard views of the whole of the spine with antero-posterior and lateral tomograms of the fractured or luxated area. At present, the unquestionable contribution of the CT. Scanner should be borne in mind, especially for the visualisation of a retropulsed osseous fragment into the spinal canal and hence in the evaluation of its diameter, as the basis of the so-called "recalibration" procedure. The assessment should give the precise information fundamental to treatment: the site and type of lesion; the notion of stability or instability which is indeed difficult to define, judging by the number of classifications, whether they be anatomical or based on the fracture mechanism. The value of contrast investigations is essentially limited to serious neurological lesions not accounted for by sufficient osteoligamentary damage, in which case the cause may be a disc herniation or an arachnoid cyst, or limited to post-operational studies to affirm the quality of the osseous situation and decompression of the spinal canal.

In 1986, thoraco-lumbar spinal traumatic lesions still present two different types: on the one hand, there are osteoligamentary lesions well-evidenced by modern investigation, notably the CT scanner, and which have benefited from the sophistication of surgical approach, in particular anterior or antero-lateral, and from osteo-synthetic materials well adapted to lesion mechanisms. On the other hand, there are spinal medullary lesions, the treatment of which remains disappointing, offering as COLLINS (1984) rightly stated, no more hope of spinal function recovery nowadays than was the case fifty years ago.

As regards treatment, there is still conflict between those in favour of conservative treatment, the indications of which are well known (FRANKEL *et al.*), and those advocating surgery at a fairly early stage. However, neither has proved to be better than the other.

In all cases, the aim is to reduce and stabilize osseous lesions, lessen the risk of complications, and facilitate rehabilitation.

We hope that in the future new grafting and transplant techniques will be possible, although their efficacy is in question at present.

ROBERT P. VIGOUROUX

# Contents

## List of Contributors

Abraham, Professor Jacob, MBBS, MS (Gen. Surg.), MS (Neuro), FACS, FACA, FAMS, C.M.C. Hospital, Vellore, India.

Albert, Dr. P., Hospital "Virgen del Rocio", Avenida Manuel Siurot, s/n., E-41013 Sevilla, Spain.

Babcock, Dr. Diane S., Department of Radiology and Pediatrics, Children's Hospital Medical Center and the University of Cincinnati College of Medicine, 111 Wellington Place, Cincinnati, OH 45219, U.S.A.

Dohrmann, Dr. George J., Section of Neurosurgery, University of Chicago Medical Center, 5841 South Maryland Avenue, Chicago, IL 60637, U.S.A.

El Masri, W. S., F.R.C.S. Ed. The Midland Spinal Injuries Centre, Institute of Orthopaedics, Oswestry, Shropshire SY10 7AG, U.K.

Firsching, Dr. R., Neurochirurgische Klinik der Universität Köln, Joseph-Stelzmann-Strasse 9, D-5000 Köln 41, Federal Republic of Germany.

Frankel, H. L., M. B., F.R.C.P., National Spinal Injuries Centre, Stoke Mandeville Hospital, Mandeville Road, Aylesbury, Bucks HP21 8AL, U.K.

Frowein, Prof. Dr. R. A., Neurochirurgische Klinik der Universität Köln, Joseph-Stelzmann-Strasse 9, D-5000 Köln 41, Federal Republic of Germany.

Hacker, Prof. Dr. H., Abteilung für Neuroradiologie, Klinikum der Johann-Wolfgang-Goethe-Universität, Theodor-Stern-Kai 7, D-6000 Frankfurt/Main 70, Federal Republic of Germany.

Köning, Dr. W., Neurochirurgische Klinik der Universität Köln, Joseph-Stelzmann-Strasse 9, D-5000 Köln 41, Federal Republic of Germany.

Kummer, Prof. Dr. B., Anatomisches Institut der Universität Köln, Josef-Stelzmann-Strasse 9, D-5000 Köln 41, Federal Republic of Germany.

McLaurin, Prof. Dr. R. L., Department of Neurosurgery, University of Cincinnati College of Medicine, 111 Wellington Place, Cincinnati, OH 45219, U.S.A.

Muñoz, Dr. M. A., Hospital "Virgen del Rocio", Avenida Manuel Siurot, s/n., E-41013 Sevilla, Spain.

Murillo, Dr. F., Hospital "Virgen del Rocio", Avenida Manuel Siurot, s/n., E-41013 Sevilla, Spain.

Ravichandran, G., M. B., F.R.C.S. Ed., Spinal Injuries Unit, Lodge Moor Hospital, Sheffield S10 4LH, U.K.

Reynier, Dr. Y., Clinique Neuro-Chirurgicale, Groupe Hospitalier de la Timone, Bd. Jean Moulin, F-13385 Marseille Cedex 5, France.

Rubin, Dr. J. M., Department of Radiology, University of Michigan Hospitals, Ann Arbor, Michigan, U.S.A.

Stauffer, Prof. Dr. E. S., Southern Illinois University School of Medicine, P.O. Box 3926, Springfield, IL 62708, U.S.A.

Tsubokawa, Prof. Dr. T., Department of Neurological Surgery, Nihon University School of Medicine, Itabashi-Ku, Tokyo, Japan.

# Epidemiology of Spinal Cord Injuries

W. KÖNING, R. A. FROWEIN, and R. FIRSCHING

Neurochirurgische Universitätsklinik, Cologne
(Federal Republic of Germany)

With 4 Figures

**Contents**



## 1. Incidence

The incidence of spinal cord injury (SCI), defined as an injury resulting in paralysis or debilitating weakness as a consequence of trauma to the spinal cord, has been statistically analyzed within the last 25 years in several countries. Epidemiological data from the medical literature from 1960 to 1978 and recent studies were compiled by J. Kraus in 1980. In his critical evaluation, he gave an account of the methodological difficulties involved due to the variability of data collection and investigations as well as to lack of uniformity of terms and definitions.

With these critical thoughts in mind, the following estimates of the incidence of SCI must be regarded with caution.

Table 1. *Numbers and Rates of Incidence of SCI Reported in Selected Studies Published in 1961–1978, Reviewed by Kraus 1980, Completed by Recent Studies up to 1985*

| Authors | Year of publ. | Location of study | Period of study | No. of cases | New cases | Exist. cases | All other |
|---|---|---|---|---|---|---|---|
| | | | | | Rate per million per year | | |
| | | | | | *D, E | C, D, E, F | |
| 1 Benes | 1968 | Czecho-slovakia | 1950–64 | 241** | 13.5*** | | |
| 2 Botterell *et al.* | 1975 | Canada | 1969–70 | 224 | 14.7 | | |
| 3 Burke | 1977 | Australia | 1966–76 | 917 | | | 23 |
| 4 Cheshire | 1968 | Australia | 1959–66 | 390 | | | 17.1 |
| 5 Gehrig-Michaelis | 1968 | Switzerland | 1963–67 | 584 | 13.3 | | |
| 6 Key-Retief | 1970 | South Africa | 1963–67 | 300 | | | 17 |
| 7 Kraus *et al.* | 1975 | California, U.S.A. | 1970–71 | 619 | 33.1 (53.4)**** | 200 | |
| 8 Sutton | 1973 | Australia | 1963–70 | 232 | | | 14.4 |
| 9 Minaire *et al.* | 1978 | France | 1970–75 | 351 | 12.7 | 250 | |
| 10 Gjone-Nordlie | 1978 | Norway | 1974–75 | 131 | 16.5 | | |
| 11 Young | 1979 | NSCIDRC, U.S.A. | 1973–77 | 615 | 30.5 | | |
| 12 Fine *et al.* | 1979 | Alabama, U.S.A. | 1973–76 | 359 | | | 29.4 |
| 13 Kalsbeek *et al.* | 1980 | HSCI-Survey, U.S.A. | 1970–74 | 1,236 | 50 | 130 | |
| 14 Bracken *et al.* | 1981 | HDS, U.S.A. | 1970–77 | 430 | 40.1 | | |
| 15 Clifton | 1983 | Houston, U.S.A. | 1981 | 183 | | | 60 |
| 16 Eng Seng Tan | 1985 | Malaysia | 1985 | 713 | 27.2 | | |
| 17 Köning-Frowein | 1985 | FRG | 1983 | 877 | 35.7 | 72 | |

* Period of treatment after accident, see page 3.
** Cases of SCI-Center, Prag.
*** Estimate based on admissions to six centers.
**** Including fatal cases.

In Table 1, numbers and average annual rates of occurrence and frequency of acute spinal cord injury are listed as compiled by Kraus 1980 (published in his Table 2). Selected studies from 1979 to 1985 are added.

To facilitate interpretation, several periods after trauma have been distinguished (Fig. 1):

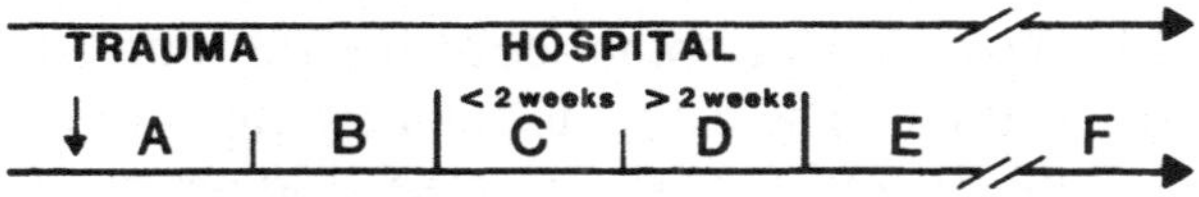


Fig. 1. Periods after trauma

A patients, dying at the scene of accident or during transportation
B patients not hospitalized with less severe spinal trauma
C patients with spinal cord injury, hospitalized for less than 2 weeks
D patients with spinal cord injury hospitalized for more than 2 weeks
E patients after treatment resulting in compensation of at least 20%
F patients after the acute stage with multiple admissions to hospital in the year of injury or later.

Period D, E, and/or C denote new cases, the total of period C, D, E and F adds up to existing cases.

From recent publications 3 types of reports can be distinguished:
— nationwide surveys
— regional studies
— data from one or more selected hospitals

### *1.1. Nationwide Surveys*

The Hospital Discharge Survey (HDS) by Bracken, Freemann, and Hellenbrand (1981) refers to the incidence of hospitalization for an acute spinal cord injury in the United States of America over an eight year period from 1970 to 1977. It is based on discharge records from randomly selected hospitals across the country according to the International Classification of Diseases, Adapted Eighth Revision (ICDA-8) codes 806 (fracture of vertebral column with spinal cord injury) and 958 (spinal cord lesion without evidence of spinal bone injury).

This study represents only new cases according to period D of our Fig. 1, eliminating the data of all patients dying before or at admission or patients not hospitalized or hospitalized for less than 15 days (period A, B, and C). Thus most patients admitted to several other hospitals before admission to the hospital of specific treatment as well as patients readmitted to hospital for recurrent complications, were not included (period F). The overall eight-year incidence was 40.1 per million population in the US (standard error = SE = 8.3).

Critical comments on this study had been published by Fine *et al.* (1982).

The National Head and Spinal Cord Injury Survey (NHSCIS) by Kalsbeek *et al.* (1980) indicates the occurrence of new cases and the frequency of existing cases for the population of the contiguous United States for the year 1974 from the National Head and Spinal Cord Injury Survey. The estimates are based on discharge records of 205 selected hospitals of 1,236 head and/or spinal cord injuries and 31 patients with spinal cord injuries alone. The estimate for new cases of SCI was 50 per million (period C, D, E), and for existing cases 130 per million population (period C, D, E, F).

The incidence rate for the Federal Republic of Germany (FRG) can be estimated as follows:

The general local health insurance, called "Allgemeine Ortskrankenkasse" (AOK) had 25.7 million persons insured in 1983. The AOK data are based partly on total counts, partly on representative counts of primary diagnoses from hospital discharge files, referring to a total number of 13.3 million persons insured at AOK.

The codes used for spinal cord injuries were about the same as those used by Bracken 1981, namely 806 and 952 of ICD, 9th Rev., 1979, corresponding to period C and D as well as readmissions (period F), excluding patients dying before or at admission to hospital (period A) and less severe not hospitalized cases (period B).

By this approach the rate of incidence for 1983 was estimated to be 66 per million of the population, which is a total of 4,065 cases per year for the FRG-population except for those cases compensated by workmen's compensation.

Workmen's compensation in the FRG is a compulsory accident insurance (Berufsgenossenschaft, BG) for 19.3 million workers and employees. Only injuries occurring at work or while commuting between place of work and home may be compensated, thus excluding injuries during time off. Only cases with a residual minimum disability to work of 20% were counted (period E).

In 1983 first-time compensation was granted in 316 cases of injury of the vertebral column with spinal cord lesions, including fatal cases (corresponding to the periods A and E of Fig. 1). The occurrence rate is 11.7 per million persons insured. Out of the total of 316 cases, 133 died (42%). This compares to the Californian study by Kraus (1975) with 294 fatalities out of 619 cases (43%).

Out of the 133 fatal cases 80% died at the site of accident. This high proportion of immediate death caused by SCI is remarkable.

The data of the central office for para- and tetraplegic patients at the SCI-Hospital, Hamburg (Meinecke 1983) is based on the hospital admissions records of 16 SCI centers throughout the FRG. The total number

Table 2. *Estimate of the Incidence of SCI for the Federal Republic of Germany (FRG) Population in 1983*

| Source | New cases | | | Existing cases | | |
|---|---|---|---|---|---|---|
| | Period after SCI (ABCDEF)* | Number per year | Rate per mill. pop. | Period after SCI (ABCDEF)* | Number per year | Rate per mill. pop. |
| 1. Central Office for Paraplegics, Hamburg | CDE | 680 | — | CDEF | 1,360 | — |
| 2.1 Workmen's Comp. | AE | 316 | 11.7 | — | — | — |
| 2.2 Workmen's Comp. | E | 183 | 6.8 | EF | 366 | 13.6 |
| 3. AOK-Data | CD | 2,030 | 33 | CDF | 4,065 | 66 |
| 4. Summ of 2.2 + 3 | CDE | 2,213 | 36 | CDEF | 4,431 | 72 |

* Period of treatment after accident, see page 3.

per year of new cases (period C and D) and existing cases (period C, D, F) was 680 and 1.360, respectively.

The ratio of new cases to existing cases was approximately 1 : 2 in 1983.

Based on the data from these three sources an estimate for the incidence of SCI of the whole population of the FRG may be made (Table 2). The incidence rate of SCI in AOK insured persons is not considered to differ from the whole population, since the age pattern and distribution of population subgroups (workers, housewives, pensioners, children) of AOK are representative for the whole population.

Since double counting of patients covered by AOK and workmen's compensation is not possible by law, 366 cases from workmen's compensation can be added to the number of 4,065 to a total of 4,431 existing cases. The estimate for new cases will be approximately 2,200 per year because the ratio of new cases to existing cases is about 1 : 2. This estimate yields an overall incidence rate of existing cases of about 72, and for new cases about 36 per million population.

### *1.2. Regional Studies*

The investigation with a complete case ascertainment of a distinct geographical area was published by Kraus in 1975 for 18 counties of northern California, including all cases, hospitalized or not, from the records from each hospital and the coroner's office throughout that area. He found an incidence of 53.4 per million of the population per year in 1970–1974. Excluding fatal cases, the incidence was 33.1 per million population.

From similarly thorough analyses Gehrig and Michaelis in Switzerland (1968) found an incidence of 13.3 per million; accordingly Gjone and Nordlie in Norway (1978) estimated the incidence to be 16.5 per million population.

### *1.3. Data from One or More Special SCI-Centers*

Being the most common type of investigation, recent data was provided by Minaire *et al.* in the Rhone-Alps region, France (1978), Fine *et al.* in Alabama, U.S.A. (1979), and Eng Seng Tan in Singapore (1985). Their data are based on hospital admissions at one specialized SCI center recruiting patients from large areas.

Recent data from several special SCI-Centers have been reported by Clifton (1983) from 3 hospitals in Texas, U.S.A., Young (1979) from 11 hospitals in Phoenix, U.S.A., and Meinecke (1984) from 16 hospitals in the FRG.

### *1.4. Discussion*

All of the frequency rates of SCI are set out in Fig. 2 for the final year of each period of study between 1950 and 1985.

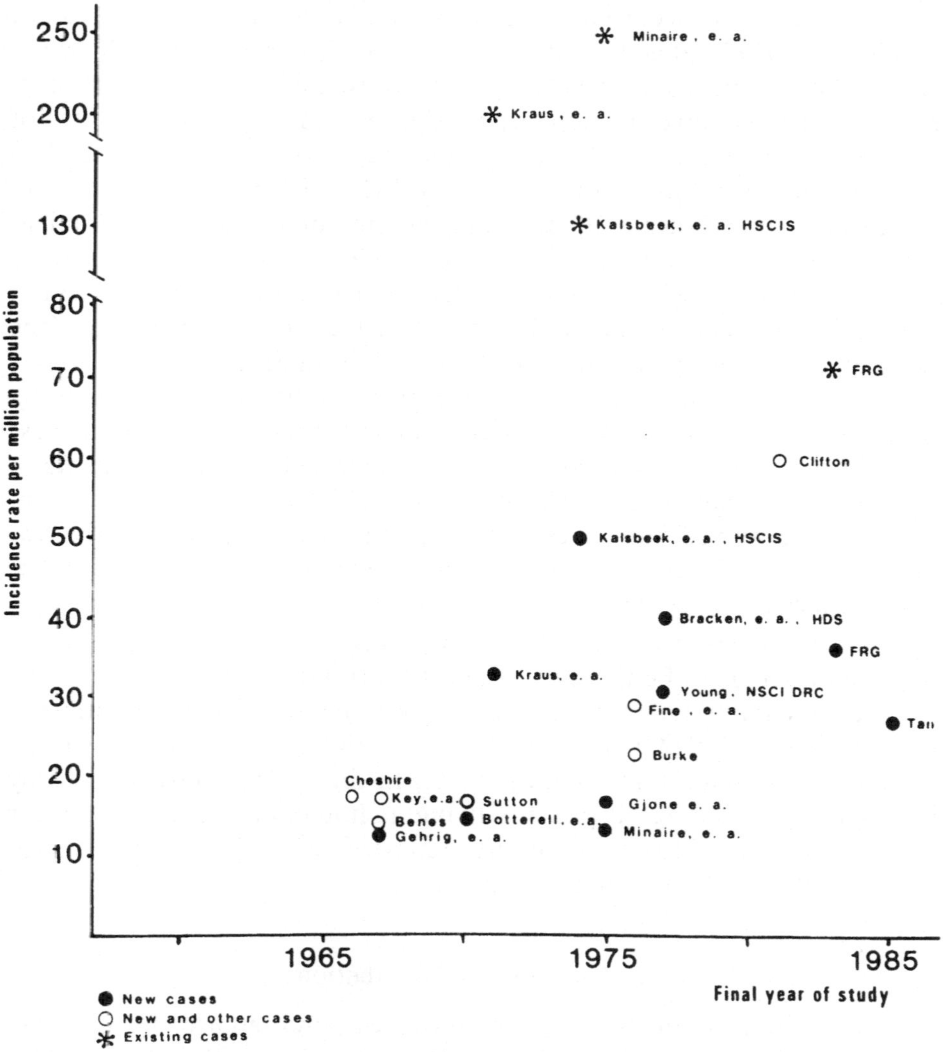


Fig. 2. Incidence rates of SCI in 1965–1985 reported in selected studies (per million population). ● new cases, ○ new cases and other, * existing cases

New cases (●), existing cases (+), and not clearly defined cases (○) are differentiated.

Although a large variation of numbers of patients is evident, a tendency towards an increasing incidence can be distinguished from 1950 to 1985, suggesting a greater need for the organization of an efficient system of management and care of spinal cord injury patients (Harris 1985, Donovan *et al.* 1984, Cheshire 1968).

From all studies, the incidence rate of 60 per million of the population as estimated by Clifton (1983) is the highest for new cases.

Estimates of the occurrence of new cases, as derived from large studies, HSCIS and HDS, range from 50 to 40.1 per million population. They are higher than estimates derived from hospital related studies. In the most extensive regional investigation, reported by Kraus *et al.* (1975) the rate of 31 new cases per million of the population is very close to our estimate of 36 cases per million of the population in the FRG in 1983.

A similar prevelance of 30 new cases per million of the population had been reported by Young (1979), based on data from 11 SCI-centers, collected by the National Spinal Cord Injury Data Research Center, NSCIDRC, Phoenix. Eng Seng Tan reported a rate of 27 per million of the population, based on data from one SCI-center in Singapore.

Most of the rates derived from earlier studies and studies using questionnaires for data collection of one or more special SCI centers are less than 20 per million of the population and are likely to be incomplete in relation to the population at risk Kurtzke (1977). A high variation of incidence is observed from investigations restricted to small areas with great differences of social economic structures as reported by Kraus *et al.* (1975) and Minaire *et al.* (1978).

Thus an occurrence rate of about 30–40 new cases per million of the population seems to be the most accurate currently.

The total amount of existing cases seems even more difficult to estimate. Rates vary from 250 (Minaire *et al.* 1978), 130 (Kalsbeek *et al.* 1980) to 71.9 per million population in our own study. In the "HIS" study (quoted by Kraus 1980) including all patients living at home, an incidence rate for existing cases of 750 per million was reported, while Kraus *et al.* (1975) found a rate of 200 per million population.

## 2. Age and Sex Distribution

The age distribution of SCI is similar to the figures reported by Kalsbeek *et al.* (1980), Kraus *et al.* (1975) and Bracken *et al.* (1980) (Fig. 3). The almost identical age specific patterns show a highest peak at the age of 15 to 24, a decreasing frequency in the middle aged groups and a second peak above the age of 55. By contrast, the almost identical figure in younger and middle aged patients showed a marked decline above the age of 55 reported by Fine *et al.* (1979). This possibly reflects the selection of patients at rehabilitation centers, which underrepresents the elderly, since they have the highest mortality rate in the acute stage (Kraus *et al.* 1975). A similar age distribution has been reported from other rehabilitation centers by Kuhn *et al.* (1983) in Switzerland, and by Clifton (1983) in Texas, U.S.A.

Age distributions with the typical 2-peak-figure are similar for each sex, the peak in males being earlier (15–24 years) than in females (25–30 years) (Fig. 4).

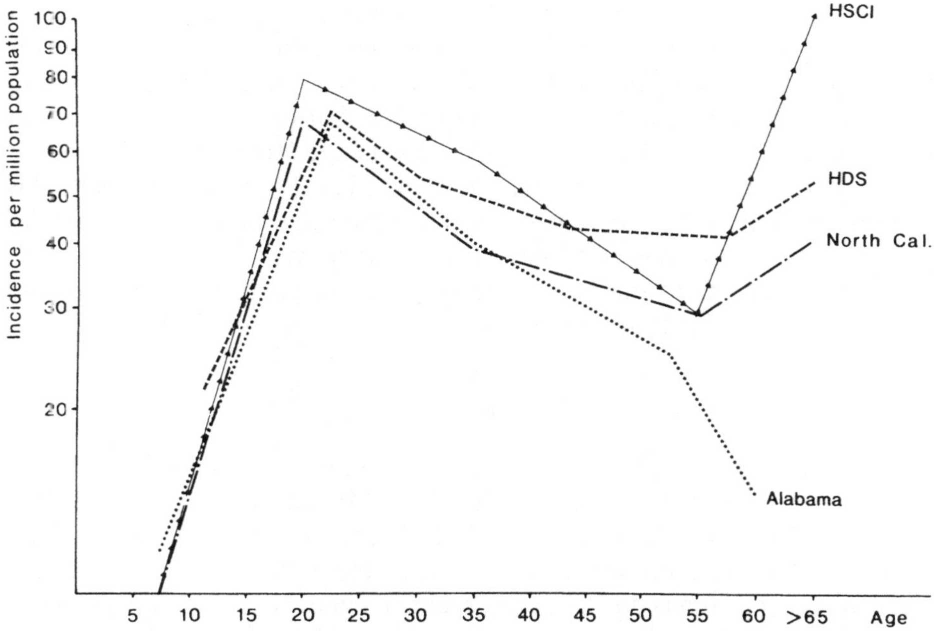


Fig. 3. Incidence rates of SCI by age (per million population) reported by Kraus *et al.* 1975, North California; Fine *et al.* 1979, Alabama; Kalsbeek *et al.* 1980, HSCIS; Bracken *et al.* 1981, HDS

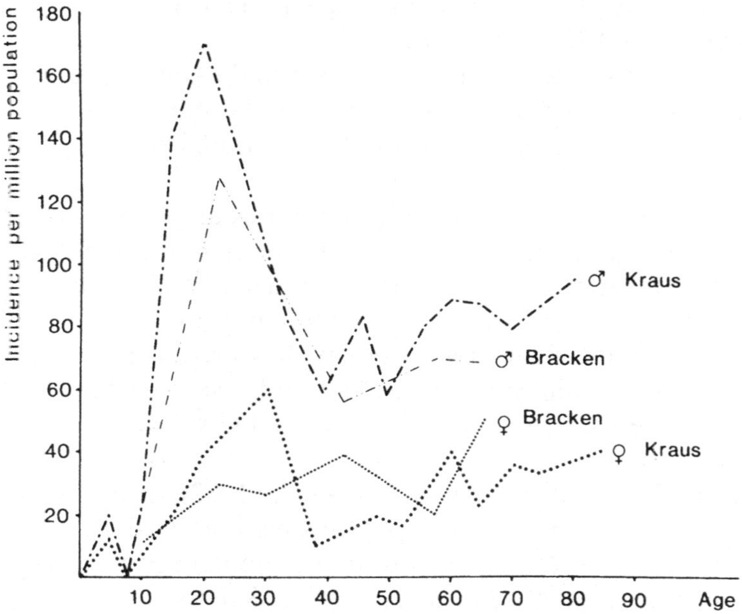


Fig. 4. Incidence rates of SCI by age and sex (per million population) reported by Kraus *et al.* 1975, Bracken *et al.* 1981

The incidence in females is remarkably lower for all age groups in most studies. By contrast, Kuhn *et al.* (1983) reported, twice the incidence rate for females below 20 years of age. Great differences in the male to female ratio have been reported: Frankel *et al.* (1968) 8.5 : 1; Sutton (1973) 7.0 : 1; Sutton *et al.* (1982) 4.3 : 1; Kuhn *et al.* (1983) 2.59 : 1; our study (1983) 2.5 : 1.

An increasing incidence in females over the last 20 years is obvious. This phenomenon may be attributed to the increasing numbers of females playing an active role in professional life and sports.

On the other hand the ratio is varying as a result of the differences in social economic, cultural and ethnical pattern (Kuhn *et al.* 1983).

## 3. Causes

A *traffic accident* is the most frequent cause of spinal cord injury in all studies (Fine *et al.* 1979, Minaire *et al.* 1978, Michaelis 1979, Clifton 1983, Eng Seng Tan 1985, Meinecke 1983). The rate of frequency ranges from 30% to 50%. Data on subgroups (motorcycle, automobile, pedestrians) vary. SCI in children is due to traffic accidents in 65% of cases (Kraus *et al.* 1975). Motorcycles and bicycles have a share of 10% to 12% (Kuhn *et al.* 1982, Fine *et al.* 1979 and 1982, Minaire *et al.* 1978). Simpson *et al.* 1981 reported that there was an excessive consumption of alcohol in one third of the accident patients who were tested.

The incidence of work related injuries ranges from 20% to 40% for all spinal cord injuries (Tator *et al.* 1984, Eng Seng Tan 1985, Ekong and Tator 1985, Meinecke 1983, Benes 1968).

In the studies by Tator and Edmonds 1979 and Ekon and Tator 1985, the rate of admissions to Sunnybrook Hospital, Toronto, SCI at work had decreased from 29.3% in the period 1948–1973 to 17.4% in the period 1974–1979.

More than 50% of the work related injuries are caused by falls from heights (Botterell *et al.* 1975), according to the findings published by Eng Seng Tan for Singapore (1985) an area of rapid industrialization for the past two decades. Falling objects are a common cause at work in mines (Guttmann 1973 and Benes 1968). Today they are less frequent.

Falls are also a main cause of accidents at home, particularly in elderly ladies falling downstairs, from chairs or ladders (Watson 1976, 1983, Michaelis 1979).

In Burma (Toe 1978) and Papua (Gee-Sinha 1982), there is a high rate of falls from trees, accounting for approximately one third of all SCI.

SCI as a result of attempted suicide by jumping from heights occurs mainly in young females (Girard *et al.* 1980, 58% less than 30 year of age and Michaelis 1979).

Sports (Hitchcock and Karmi 1982) and recreational injuries have been reported to cause SCI in 7% (Kraus *et al.* 1975); 7.5% (Minaire *et al.* 1978); (Frankel *et al.* 1969); 9% (Meinecke 1984) and 15.4% (Ekong and Tator 1985).

Among sport and recreational accidents causing SCI, diving is involved to a varying extent: 6.2% (Frankel *et al.* 1969), 14% (Sutton 1973) and in contrast 65% (Botterell *et al.* 1975), 60% (Tator *et al.* 1984) and even 75% (Kraus *et al.* 1975). Albrand and Corkill (1976) called it a summer epidemic situation for the Californian-region.

Some spinal cord injuries occur whilst playing football (5%, Sances *et al.* 1984), trampoline (Torg and Das 1985), wrestling (Gehrig and Michaelis 1968, Müller and Blyth 1982, Kewalrhami *et al.* 1980), gymnastics, break dancing (Norman and Grodin 1984), hockey (Tator and Edmonds 1984), hang-gliding (Tongue 1977), rugby (Hoskins 1979) and horseback riding (Bruce *et al.* 1984, Kuhn *et al.* 1983).

Some reports indicated a high incidence of gunshot wounds (Mc Collough *et al.* 1981, South Florida: 40%, Fine *et al.* 1976, Alabama: 20%, Clifton 1983, Texas: 25%. Jacobson and Bors 1970), and stab wounds (Peacock *et al.* 1977) reflecting regional variations (US, Vietnam war, South Africa).

## 4. Level and Functional Impairment

Paraplegia and paraparesis were slightly more frequent in the series of Fine *et al.* 1979 and Frankel *et al.* 1969, 52% and 62% respectively, tetraplegia and tetraparesis were more common in the reports by Tator *et al.* (1984) and Young (1979), 56% and 54% respectively.

The thoracolumbar junction (T 11–L 1) is affected in about 50% of all thoracic and lumbar lesions (Sances *et al.* 1984, Lifeso *et al.* 1985, Frankel *et al.* 1969, Tator *et al.* 1984, Watson 1976).

The incidence of a complete transverse section syndrome was less common in lumbar (19%), than in thoracic lesions (74%), Fine *et al.* (1982).

Some causes of injury are strongly related to the extent of lesions as reported by Kraus *et al.* 1975. Tetraparesis in particular was linked to recreational accidents (mostly diving injuries) and paraplegia to gun shot wounds (Clifton 1983, Fine *et al.* 1976, Mc Collough *et al.* 1981).

Motorvehicle accidents have been reported to cause all types of spinal neural impairment, falls mostly result in paraparesis and to a lesser extent tetraparesis (Kraus *et al.* 1975).

## 5. Conclusions

In evaluating the relevance of the incidence rates of SCI reported in the literature, a very important distinction has to be made between those derived from large regional studies or survey studies, which include data from hospital admissions or discharge records from all types of hospitals, e.g., the North California study, the HDS, the HSCI survey and our own study of the FRG, and those incidence rates derived from hospital admissions of one or more special SCI centers (e.g., the studies of Gehrig and Michaelis, Gjone and Nordlie, Minaire *et al.*, Botterell *et al.*, Eng Seng Tan (Table 1 and Fig. 2).

Thus the incidence rate of about 30–40 per million population per year indicates the realistic number of new cases, which affects all hospitals concerned in the management of the acute phase of SCI. For planning the long term care the relevant incidence rate of new cases is about 20 per million population per year, because not all of the fatal cases nor all of the cases with lesser or transient neurological impairment nor all of the elderly patients reach the special SCI center.

The age distribution of acute SCI has the highest peak in the age-group of 15 to 24. This is a constant finding in all studies. In the groups of existing cases the number of older patients is increasing as reported by Eisenberg and Tierney (1985) who analyzed data from the Veterans Administration.

For modern industrial countries with a high traffic density some trends can be stated:

— more than 50% of all SCI are caused by traffic accidents,
— there is an increasing number of injuries to females and of sport-related injuries and
— a decreasing number of industrial-related SCI.

## 6. Summary

The medical literature of the epidemiology of the spinal cord injuries published in the past 20 years are reviewed.

A great study related variation of the annual incidence rates can be stated ranging from 12.7 to 50 per million population for new cases and from 72–250 per million population for existing cases. Different methods of investigation, different periods of study and different social economic structures of the population are possible explanations.

A general agreement was found between the results from the HSCI-Survey, the HDS, the North California Study and from our own FRG-Study, which is about 30–40 per million population.

Other epidemiological data as age and sex distribution, cause and level of injury are compiled by the literature.

## References

1. Albrand OW, Corkill G (1976) Broken necks from diving accidents. Am J Sports Med 4 (3): 107 – 110
2. AOK-Bundesverband (Krankheitsartenstatistik 1983), Bonn (Germany), FRG, 1985

3. Benes V (1968) Spinal cord injury. Baillière, Tindall and Cassell, London
4. Botterell EH, Jousse AT, Kraus AS, Thompson MG (1975) A model for the future care of acute spinal cord injuries. Can J Neurol Sci 2 (4): 361 – 380
5. Bracken MB, Freeman DH, Hellenbrand K (1981) Incidence of acute traumatic hospitalized spinal cord injury in the United States, 1970–1977. Am J Epidemiol 113 (6): 615 – 622
6. Bruce DA, Schut L, Sutton LN (1984) Brain and cervical spine injuries occurring during organized sports activities in children and adolescents. Primary Care vol 11 Nr 1 pp 175 – 194
7. Burke DC (1977) Spinal cord injuries. Aust NZ J Surg 47: 166 – 170
8. Cheshire DJ (1968) The complete and centralised treatment of paraplegia. Paraplegia 6: 59 – 73
9. Clifton GL (1983) Spinal cord injury in the Houston-galveston area. Tex Med 79 (9): 55 – 57
10. Donovan WH, Carter RE, Bedbrook GM *et al.* (1984) Incidence of medical complications in spinal cord injury: patients in specialised, compared with non-specialised centers. Paraplegia 22 (5): 282 – 290
11. Eisenberg MG, Tierney DO (1985) Changing demographic profile of the spinal cord injury population: Implications for health care support systems. Paraplegia 23: 335 – 343
12. Eng Seng Tan (1985) The care of paraplegics and tetraplegics. Paraplegia 23: 159 – 163
13. Ekong CE, Tator CH (1985) Spinal cord injury in the work force. Can J Surg 28 (2): 165 – 167
14. Fine PR, Stafford MA, Miller JM, Stover SL (1976) Gunshot wounds of the spinal cord: a survey of literature and epidemiologic study of 48 lesions in Alabama. Ala J Med Sci 13 (2): 173 – 180
15. Fine PR, Kuhlemeier KV, De Vivo MJ, Stover SL (1979) Spinal cord injury: an epidemiologic perspective. Paraplegia 17 (2): 237 – 250
16. Fine PR, De Vivo MJ, Mc Eachran AG (1982) Incidence of acute traumatic hospitalized spinal cord injury in the United States, 1970–1977. Am J Epidemiol 115 (3): 475 – 479
17. Frankel HL, Hancock DO, Hyslop G, Melzak J, Michaelis LS, Ungar GH, Vernon JDS, Walsh JJ (1969) The value of postural reduction in the initial management of closed injuries of the spine with paraplegia and tetraplegia. Paraplegia 7: 179 – 192
18. Gee RW, Sinha SN (1982) The epidemiology of spinal cord injuries in Papua New Guinea. Papua New Guinea Med J 25 (2): 97 – 99
19. Gehrig R, Michaelis LS (1968) Statistics of acute paraplegia and tetraplegia on a national scale. Switzerland 1960–1967. Paraplegia 6: 93 – 95
20. Girard R, Minaire P, Castanier M, Berard E, Perrineriche B (1980) Spinal cord injury by falls. Paraplegia 18: 381 – 385.
21. Gjone R, Nordlie L (1978) Incidence of traumatic paraplegia and tetraplegia in Norway: a statistical survey of the years 1974 and 1975. Paraplegia 16 (1): 88 – 93.
22. Guttmann L (1973) Spinal cord injuries. Blackwell, Oxford London Edinburgh Melbourne.

23. Harris P (1985) Acute spinal cord injury patients—who cares? Paraplegia 23: 1 – 7
24. Hitchcock ER, Karmi MZ (1982) Sports injuries to the central nervous system. JR Coll Surg Edinb 27 (1): 46 – 49
25. Hoskins T (1979) Rugby injuries to the cervical spine in English schoolboys. Practitioner 223 (1335): 365 – 366
26. Jacobson SA, Bors E (1970) Spinal cord injury in Vietnamese combat. Paraplegia 7 (4): 263 – 281
27. Kalsbeek WD, Mc Laurin RL, Harris BS, Miller JD (1980) The national head and spinal cord injury survey: major findings. J Neurosurg (Suppl) 53: 19 – 31
28. Kewalramani LS, Kraus JF, Sterling HM (1980) Acute spinal-cord lesions in a pediatric population: Epidemiological and clinical features. Paraplegia 18 (3): 206 – 219
29. Key AG, Retief PJ (1970) Spinal cord injuries. An analysis of 300 new lesions. Paraplegia 7: 243 – 249
30. Kraus JF, Franti CE, Riggins RS, Richards D, Borhani NO (1975) Incidence of traumatic spinal cord lesions. J Chronic Dis 28 (9): 471 – 492
31. Kraus JF (1980) Injury to the head and spinal cord. The epidemiological relevance of the medical literature published from 1960 to 1978. J Neurosurg (Suppl.) 53: 3 – 10
32. Kraus JF (1980) A comparison of recent studies on the extent of the head and spinal cord injury problem in the United States. J Neurosurg (Suppl) 53: 35 – 43
33. Kuhn H, Zaech GA, Koechlin P, Urwyler A (1983) Comparison of spinal cord injuries in females and in males, 1979 – 1981, Basle. Paraplegia 21 (3): 154 – 160
34. Kurtzke JF (1977) Epidemiology of spinal cord injury. Neurol Neurochir Psiquiatr 18 (2 – 3 Suppl): 187 – 191
35. Lifeso RM, Arabie KM, Kadhi SKM (1985) Fractures of the thoraco-lumbar spine. Paraplegia 23: 207 – 224
36. McCollough III NC, Green BA, Klose KJ, Goldberg ML, Klose C (1981) Spinal cord injury in South Florida. J. Florida MA 68 (12): 968 – 973
37. Meinecke FW (1983) BG-Central office for paraplegic patients. Die BG, 1. Erich Schmidt Verlag GmbH, Bielefeld, pp 1 – 7
38. Meinecke FW (1984) Primary treatment of paraplegic patients. Unfallchirurgie 10: 152 – 158
39. Michaelis LS (1979) Epidemiology of spinal cord injury. In: Vinken PJ, Bruyn GW, Braakman R (eds) Handbook of clinical neurology, vol 25, 2. North-Holland Publishing Comp, Amsterdam Oxford, American Elsevier Publishing Co, New York, pp 141 – 143
40. Minaire P, Castanier M, Girard R, Berard E, Deidier C, Bourret J (1978) Epidemiology of spinal cord injury in the Rhone-Alps Region, France, 1970 – 1975. Paraplegia 16 (1): 76 – 87
41. Mueller F, Blyth C (1982) Epidemiology of sports injuries in children. Clinics in Sports Medicine 1 (3): 343 – 352
42. Norman RA, Grodin MA (1984) Injuries from break dancing. Am Fam Physician 30 (4): 109 – 112

43. Peacock WJ, Shrosbree RD, Key AG (1977) A review of 450 stabwounds of the spinal cord. S Afr Med J 51 (26): 961 – 964
44. Sances A, Mykelbust JB, Maiman DJ, Larson SJ, Cusick JF, Jodat RW (1984) The biomechanics of spinal injuries. In: Bourne, JR (ed), Critical reviews in biomechical engineering, vol 11 (1) CRC Press, Boca Raton, Florida
45. Selecki BR, Ring IT, Simpson DA, Vanderfield GK, Sewell MF (1982) Trauma to the central and peripheral nervous systems: Part I: an overview of mortality, morbidity and costs: NSW 1977. Aust NZ J Surg 52 (1): 93 – 102
46. Simpson D, Antonio JD, North JB, Ring IT, Selecki BR, Sewell MF (1981) Fatal injries of the head and spine: epidemiological studies in New South Wales and South Australia. Med J Aust 2 (12 – 13): 660 – 664
47. Sutton NG (1973) Injuries of the spinal cord: The management of paraplegia and tetraplegia. Butterworths, London
48. Sutton RA, Bentley M, Castree B, Mattinson R, Pattinson J, Smith R (1982) Review of the social situation of paraplegic and tetraplegic patients rehabilitated in the Hexham Regional Spinal Injury Unit in the North of England over the past four years. Paraplegia 20: 71 – 79
49. Tator CH, Edmonds VE (1979) Acute spinal cord injury: analysis of epidemiologic factors. Can J Surg 22 (6): 575 – 578
50. Tator CH, Rowed DW, Schwartz ML, Gertzbein SD, Bharatwal N, Barkin M, Edmonds VE (1984) Management of acute spinal cord injuries. Can J Surg 27 (3): 289 – 293
51. Tator CH, Edmonds VE (1984) National survey of spinal injuries in hockey players. Can Med Assoc J 130 (7): 875 – 880
52. Toe T (1978) Spinal injuries in Rangoon, Burma. Paraplegia 16 (1): 118 – 120
53. Tongue JR (1977) Hang gliding injuries in California. J Trauma 17 (12): 898 – 902
54. Torg JS, Das M (1985) Trampoline and minitrampoline injuries to the cervical spine. Clin Sports Med 4 (1): 45 – 60
55. Watson N (1976) Pattern of spinal cord injury in the elderly. Paraplegia 14 (1): 36 – 40
56. Watson N (1983) Spinal cord injury in the female. Paraplegia 21 (3): 143 – 148
57. Young JS (1979) Spinal cord injury: Associated general trauma and medical complications. In: Thompson RA, Green JR (eds) Advances in neurology, vol 22. Raven Press, New York, pp 255 – 260

# Biomechanics of the Thoracic and Lumbar Spine

B. KUMMER

Anatomisches Institut der Universität Cologne
(Federal Republic of Germany)

With 6 Figures

**Contents**



## 1. Normal Biomechanics

Normal biomechanics of the spine is characterized by the fact that several joints must be balanced at the same time. Between any two adjacent vertebrae, the equilibrium in the intervertebral disc and the joints of the vertebral arches is to be maintained by muscular forces, a phenomenon which is repeated at the level of every segment of mobility. In the normal upright posture, the gravity centers of the different parts of the body lie in front of the vertebral column, causing forwardly directed torques which must be counteracted by the backwardly directed torques of the dorsal musculature. The total load of any segment of the spine is therefore given by the resultant from (partial) body weight and muscle force.

The form of the entire vertebral column is, furthermore, controlled by the play of antagonistic muscle groups. The contraction of the dorsal muscles accentuates the lordosis and straightens the kyphosis; contraction of the ventral muscles (M. rectus abdominis), on the other hand, amplifies the kyphosis and straightens the lordosis. Since, in most positions of the body, the ventral muscles act synergetically with the body weight, the total load either of a few segments or of the whole compartment of the spine is increased by their contraction.

The resultant of all forces acting on any segment of the vertebral column is the vector sum of body weight and muscle forces (Fig. 1). Its action line

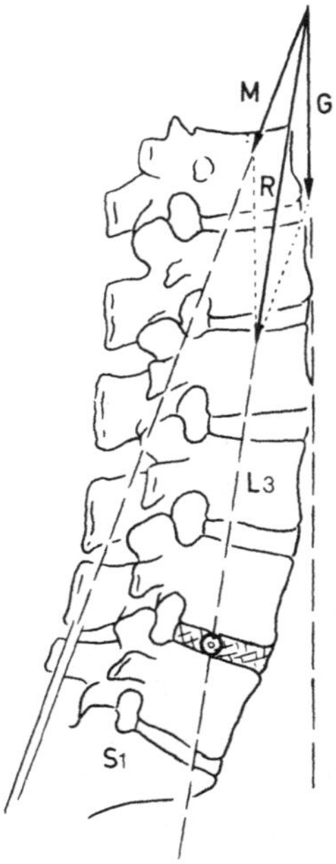


Fig. 1

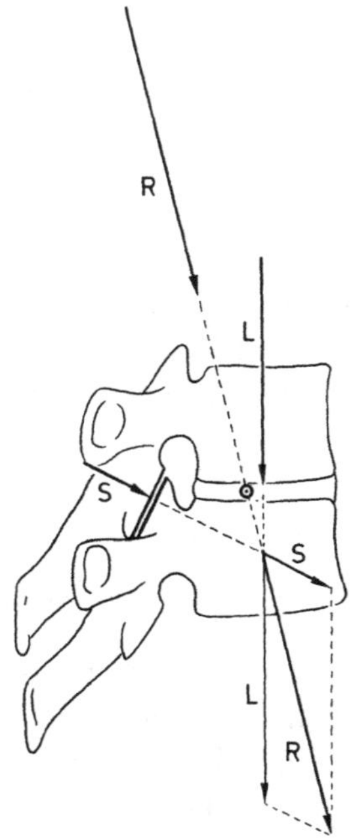


Fig. 2

Fig. 1. Construction of the resultant force, stressing the junction between lumbar 4 and 5. *G* body weight, *L 3* third lumbar vertebra, *M* muscle force, *R* resultant of the forces G and M, *S 1* first sacral vertebra

Fig. 2. Stresses on the intervertebral joint. The resultant force *R* (see Fig. 1) can be split into the longitudinal force *L* (perpendicular to the plane of the disc) and the force *S*, perpendicular to the articular surface

runs exactly through the center of rotation, and, therefore, the total torque is zero. The rotational center is not exactly defined; it is situated somewhere inside the intervertebral disc, in most cases close to the center of the nucleus pulposus.

The resultant of forces is not necessarily perpendicular to the surface of the vertebral body; it can be split into a normal and a tangential (shear) component. The normal component represents the pressure between the adjoining vertebrae, while the tangential component tends to dislocate the upper vertebra ventrally. A true dislocation is, however, prevented by the fibrous ring of the disc and by the joints of the arch (Fig. 2). As a result, the intervertebral disc is under stress by compression and shear, while the articular facets have to withstand pure compression (see Kummer 1983).

The compressive force acting on the upper articular facet is directed ventrally, while the force on the lower facet acts in a dorsal direction (Fig. 3). This results in relatively high stresses for the interarticular portion of the vertebral arch (Schlüter 1965).

The movements of the vertebral column are limited by the fibrous ring of the intervertebral disc and by the shape and position of the vertebral joints.

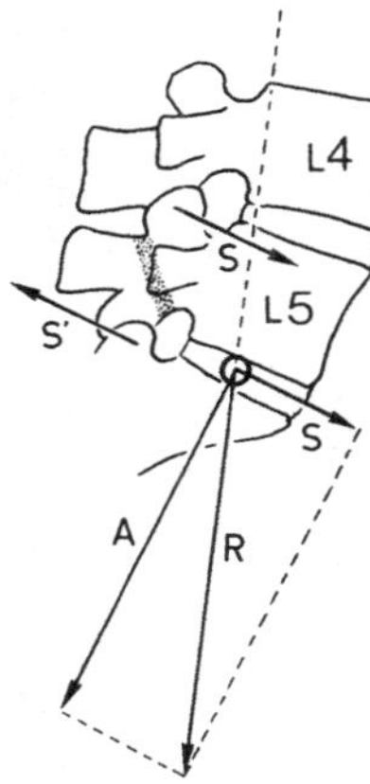


Fig. 3. The interarticular portion of the arch (stippled) is stressed by the forces *S* and *S'*. *A* axial force (relative to *L 5*), *L 4* and *L 5* fourth and fifth lumbar vertebrae, *R* resultant force, *S* ventrally shifting component of *R*, *S'* resistance at lumbo-sacral junction (equal magnitude, but opposite direction as *S*)

In the thoracic spine, rotation and ventral bending are relatively free, lateral flexion and extension are restricted. Especially the narrow spaces between the laminae and between the spinous processes are limiting factors for dorsal flexion (extension).

The lumbar spine is characterized by the freedom of dorsal and ventral flexion, restricted lateral flexion and minimal rotational movements (c.f., Kummer 1981, Putz 1976).

Lateral flexion is possible especially in the thoraco-lumbar and lumbo-sacral junctions.

No precisely fixed axes for these movements exist. This is mainly due to the complex structure of the intervertebral disc. It behaves like an elastic cushion and, therefore, has no defined center of rotation.

However, the axis for lateral rotation in the thoracic spine seems to be

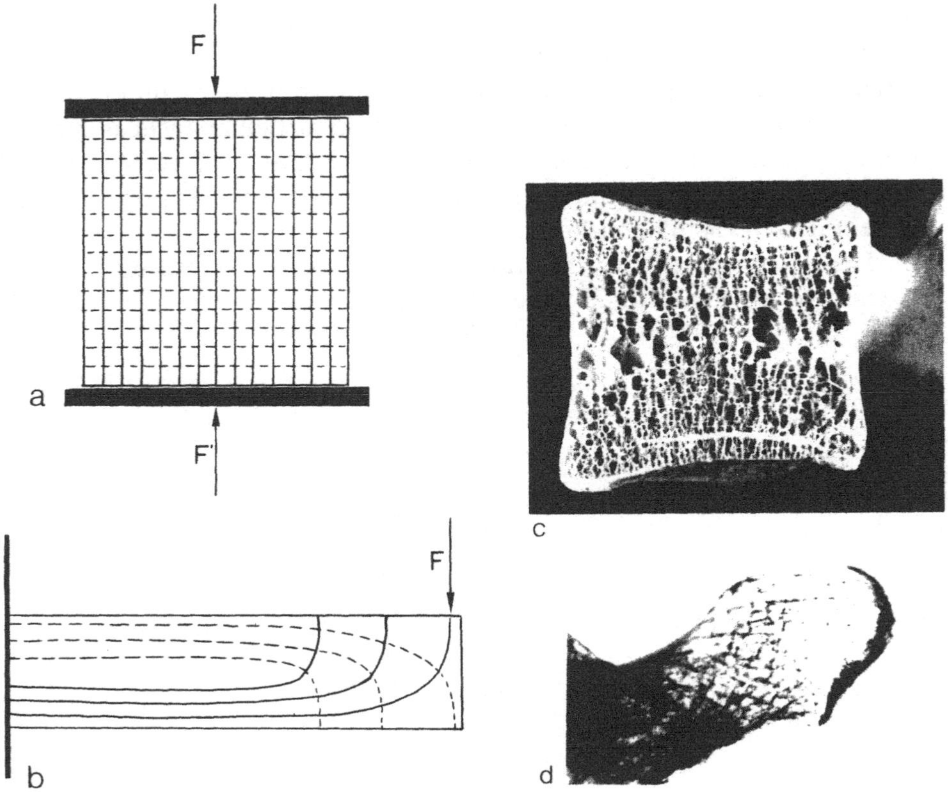


Fig. 4. a) Trajectorial pattern, characteristic for pure compression stress. *F* and *F'* compressive force and counterforce, solid lines = compressive stress trajectories, interrupted lines = tensile stress trajectories. b) Stress trajectories in a beam under bending stress (legend to symbols corresponds to Fig. 4a). c) Sagittal section through a lumbar vertebral body, the spongy elements reflect the trajectorial pattern of compression stress. d) Radiograph of a thoracic transverse process. The pattern of the spongy bone is similar to the arrangement of stress trajectories in a beam, stressed by bending (see Fig. 4b)

localized in the posterior part of the vertebral body or in the vertebral channel, respectively.

The internal structure of the vertebra is adapted to its mechanical stress. The spongious architecture of the vertebral body exactly reflects the trajectorial pattern, characteristic for axial compression (c.f., Kummer 1982), while the spinous processes in the different parts of the vertebral column are stressed either by axial compression or by bending, respectively (see Kummer 1960). The transverse processes of the thoracic spine are generally subjected to bending stresses, which is expressed clearly in the pattern of their spongy bone (Fig. 4).

## 2. Biomechanics of Traumatism

Traumatic destruction of the vertebral column can be caused by:
a) an abnormal quantity of stress
b) an abnormal quality of stress
c) a combination of a) and b)

*An abnormal quantity of stress* means that the direction and position of the resultant force are normal or nearly normal, but that the magnitude of the force exceeds the breaking strength of the material. The term "abnormality" in this context is relative; it describes the relationship between the resistance of the tissues (bone and ligaments) and the actual magnitude of forces. Therefore, "abnormal quantity of stresses" is also given by a "normal" load, acting on an osteoporotic bone.

Trauma by overloading of the vertebral column causes (more or less) axial compression of the vertebral bodies without dislocation. The height of the damaged vertebral body decreases, but the strength of its spongy bone increases with increasing compression. Plaue (1973) described the almost complete regain of the initial strength after compression of the vertebral bodies to 50% of their former height.

Compression fracture of the vertebral body is only rarely followed by rupture of the annulus fibrosus. In Brinckmann's (1985) experiments, no herniation of disc material was ever observed. From this, it may be concluded that injury of the thoracic or lumbar discs is, in most cases, related to a structural deficiency of the latter.

*Abnormal stress quality* refers to deviation of the resultant force from its normal position and direction. In trauma, it is generally caused by a considerable external force, which usually overshadows all other forces, as for example body weight and muscle forces, so that it is almost identical with the resultant. The skeleton and the articular ligaments are extremely weak in counteracting abnormally directed loads, because of their functional adaptation to the normal types of load.

The destructive potential of the external force is given by the torque, i.e. the force, multiplied by its lever arm. This is important, especially for *transverse forces*, which cause bending or torsional moments. In both cases, the destructive effect begins when the limits of the normal range of motion are reached.

Dorsally directed bending moments are extremely dangerous, because the extension of the spine is limited by the joints of the arches and, in the thoracic compartment, by the contact of the spinous processes (Veleanu *et al.* 1972). This type of stress may cause fractures of the pedicles and of the vertebral body by compression of its dorsal part.

Extreme ventral bending results in tensile stresses on interspinous ligaments, the ligamenta flava and the capsules of the vertebral joints and in compression stresses on the intervertebral discs and the ventral parts of the vertebral bodies. The weakest part in this construction is generally the spongy bone of the vertebral body. Ventral compression fractures may result.

Lateral bending results in bending stress for the vertebral body, i.e. compression on the concave side of the bend and tension on the convex side. Destruction often begins on the tension side.

Torsional moments primarily stress the intervertebral discs and, especially in the lumbar spine, the vertebral joints. They produce ruptures of the fibers of the annulus fibrosus as well as fractures of the articular processes.

Every extreme movement of the spine is braced, step by step, beginning at the segments with the smallest range of motion. This is the reason why the thoraco-lumbar transition is especially threatened in the case of extreme bending moments. The movement continues in this segment even when all other segments of motion are already braced by the ligaments or by the terminal positions of their joints. The rest of the spine may now be compared with a rigid lever, upon which the damaging force acts. A very high stress at the level of this junction is the result.

Injuries are not caused exclusively by external forces, but also by inertial forces of the body mass itself. Acceleration or deceleration may be responsible for considerable moments due to the potential energy of parts of the body. Bending and torsional moments can originate by this process, as well as by the influence of external forces.

A special type of stress is shearing stress, due to the horizontal component of an oblique resultant force (c.f., part 1, p. 18). This is resisted primarily by the interarticular portion of the arch, and the intervertebral disc is under stress by this force only after that part of the arch is fractured.

Fractures of this type are, however, not usually caused by extreme instantaneous stresses but by chronic overloading. The lower lumbar segments are especially exposed to this danger. This is at least one of the causes of spondylolisthesis (Schlüter 1965).

## 3. Biomechanics of Osteosyntheses

The fixation of smaller or larger segments of the spine can be performed by means of autoplastic or alloplastic osteosyntheses.

The autoplastic material (bone graft) is very sensitive to inadequate loading. In particular, bending stress causes paradox bone resorption, followed by collapse of the graft.

According to Pauwels (1971) the principle of successful bone-grafting consists in positioning the graft at sites where it is under stress by axial forces and not by bending. In practice, this means, that the graft should be applied on the tension side of the bending stresses (Fig. 5). For the spine, however, it is difficult to localize general zones of tension and compression of bending, because it can be bent to opposite sides, forwards and backwards, to the left and to the right. The graft will, therefore, be subjected to bending stresses in any position. This explains, why bone grafts are so often weakened by resorptive processes.

The mechanical solution to the problem consists in creating circum-

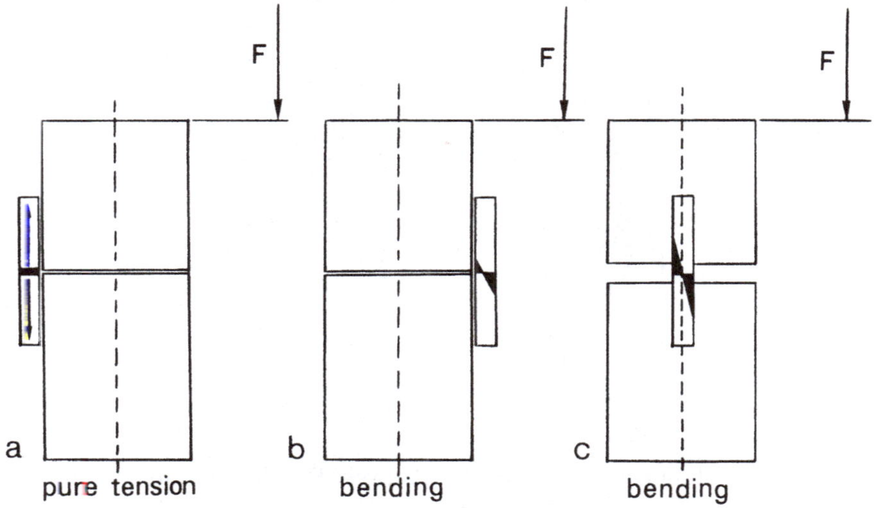


Fig. 5. Pauwels' explanation of the stresses in a bone graft. a) Position on the tensile side of the bending: the graft is stressed by tension alone. b) Position on the compression side of the bending: the graft is stressed by bending. c) Position in the middle of a relatively wide cleft: the graft is stressed by bending. *F* eccentric force. The stress diagram in every graft is marked by the dark color. Stresses which are directed upwards are positive (tension), while those directed downwards are negative (compression)

stances, under which the graft is stressed by compression only. This can be done when the spine is flexed forwards and one or two grafts are squeezed between two laminae or, preferably, between spinous processes. But, even with this technique, it is difficult to avoid any bending stress, if the graft is firmly fixed at both ends.

Pauwels, therefore, used a mobile fixation of one strong graft, squeezed between two spinous processes (Fig. 6). The mobile beds of the graft behave like joints and the graft is allowed to follow the minimal changes in direction of the resultant force, due to the changing loading of the spine. The graft is finally oriented exactly in the direction of the resultant force and bony consolidation, without any resorption, therefore occurs.

The same arguments hold for the application of alloplastic material for osteosyntheses. Repeated bending stress causes fatigue fractures, even of strong screws or plates, and, here again, it is very difficult, if not impossible, to find any localization where bending stresses never occur, even when the joints of the laminae are blocked. Harrington rods are very similar in their mechanical function to the "pendulum graft" used by Pauwels. Since they are clasped to the laminae, almost pure axial forces are transmitted to the rods. These forces are compression or tension forces, the type of stress depending on the mode of application of the clasps.

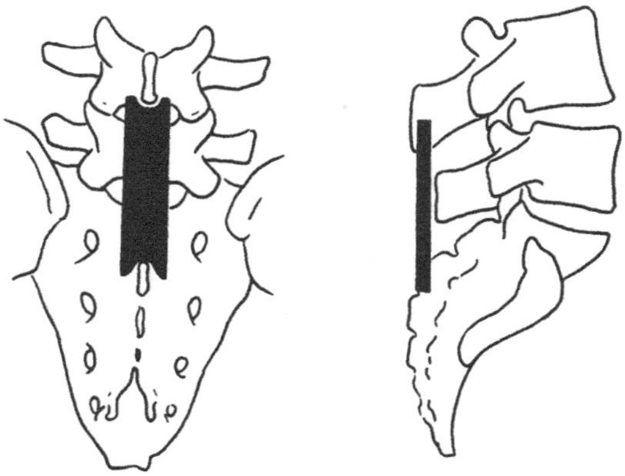

Fig. 6. The "pendulum graft", used by Pauwels for the immobilization in the lumbo-sacral transition

Paired Harrington rods provide a very solid fixation for the spine, especially when applied as tensile rods. The firmness of the fixation, however, depends on the fact, that the bridged compartment of the spine is under extreme extension. The tensile Harrington rod is, for this reason, the ideal fixation for the thoracic spine. In the lumbar spine, there may be a problem because of the danger of hyperlordosis. In this part of the vertebral column, the combination of tensile rods and interspinous bone grafts should, for mechanical reasons, be considered.

**References**

1. Brinckmann P (1985) Injury of the annulus fibrosus and disc protrusions, an in vitro investigation on human lumbar motion segments. Orthopädische Universitätsklinik Münster, Mitteilungen aus der Abteilung Biomechanik, Nr 22, April 1985
2. Kummer B (1960) Beziehungen zwischen der mechanischen Funktion und dem Bau der Wirbelsäule bei quadrupeden Säugetieren. Z Tierzücht Züchtungsbiol 74: 159 – 167
3. Kummer B (1981) Biomechanik der Wirbelgelenke. In: Die Wirbelsäule in Forschung und Praxis, Bd 87. Hippokrates, Stuttgart, pp 29 – 34

4. Kummer B (1982) Funktionelle und pathologische Anatomie der Lendenwirbelsäule. Orthop Praxis 18: 84–90
5. Kummer B (1983) Welchen Beitrag leisten die Wirbelbogengelenke zur Tragfunktion der Wirbelsäule? 5. Münch Symp exp Orthopädie: Biomechanik der Wirbelsäule. Thieme, Stuttgart, pp 19–24
6. Pauwels F (1971) Biomechanis of bone grafting. Acta Orthop Belg 37: 701–725; also in: Pauwels F, Biomechanics of the locomotor apparatus. Springer, Berlin Heidelberg New York 1980
7. Plaue R (1973) Experimentelle Untersuchungen zur funktionellen Wirbelbruchbehandlung. Monatsschr Unfallheilk 76: 395–402
8. Putz R (1976) Zur Morphologie und Rotationsmechanik der kleinen Gelenke der Lendenwirbel. Z Orthop 114: 902–912
9. Schlüter K (1965) Form und Struktur des normalen und des pathologisch veränderten Wirbels. Die Wirbelsäule in Forschung und Praxis, Bd 30. Hippokrates, Stuttgart
10. Veleanu, Grün V, Diaconescu M, Cocota E (1972) Structural peculiarities of the thoracic spine, their functional significance. Acta Anat 82: 97–107

# Clinical Aspects of Thoracic and Lumbar Spine and Spinal Cord Injuries

E. S. STAUFFER

Southern Illinois University, School of Medicine, Springfield, Illinois (U.S.A.)

## Contents

Injuries to the spine range in severity from muscle strains and ligament sprains to fracture of the vertebral bodies, fractures of the dorsal elements, dislocation of the facets, and complex combination fracture dislocations. The spinal cord and nerve roots traversing the spinal canal and neural foramina may be injured by any encroachment into the spinal canal. Patients with stable compression fractures may suffer concomitant injury to the spinal cord, and patients with grossly unstable comminuted fractures may escape neurological injury. Both of these situations, however, are relatively rare. In general, the more comminuted, displaced, and unstable the spinal fracture, the greater the likelihood of severe cord damage.

Direct injuries to the spine and spinal cord may occur by a direct blow, such as from a falling tree or other heavy object, a knife stab wound, or a missile from a gunshot. Most injuries, however, are caused by indirect trauma to the vertebral column secondary to energy generated by forces applied to the head, shoulders, trunk, or pelvis. These forces may contain an axial load as the main force with various elements of lateral bending, forward flexion, backward extension, or torsion. The thoracic and lumbar spine are most commonly injured by the kinetic energy of the person's body flying through space and coming to a sudden deceleration by hitting the shoulders, upper trunk, or buttocks against an immovable object (either by being thrown out of an automobile or from a fall from a height), and the vector of forces in a high energy bending moment become concentrated in the area of the thoracic or lumbar spine. Although injuries can occur at any level of the thoracic and lumbar spine, the most common area is at the thoracolumbar junction with specific patterns of body fracture and dorsal element dislocations at T-11–T-12, rotational flexion fractures of both body and dorsal elements at T-12–L-1, and burst fractures of the body of L-1. Fractures of the mid-thoracic spine cluster around T-5–T-6.

A specific pattern of flexion distraction injury occurs when a person is retained in a seatbelt and suffers a sudden deceleration in an automobile or airplane crash with the kinetic energy of the upper trunk and torso, causing sudden flexion and distraction centered at the mid-lumbar spine around the fulcrum of the seatbelt on the anterior abdominal wall. These commonly occur at L-2 or L-3. The fracture occurs through the dorsal spinous process and lamina and continues anteriorly through the body. The superior and inferior fragments are separated but are rarely displaced significantly in the sagittal or coronal plane. Patients with these fractures often escape spinal cord or cauda equina damage, and the fracture may be missed in the face of concomitant head injury or associated small intestine injury. Any person complaining of pain after an automobile accident while wearing a seat belt must be specifically examined for the presence of a spinal fracture.

## 1. Specific Injuries of the Thoracic Spine: Anatomy

The thoracic spine is relatively well protected from excessive displacement from injury by the rib cage, the sternum, and the enclosed chest contents. The ribs and sternum permit little flexion and extension motion of the upper and mid-thoracic spine, however, the coronal configuration of the facets allow for normal rotation motion. The facet joint angle changes abruptly at the thoracolumbar junction, usually at the dorsal element of the 12th thoracic vertebra, which has coronal shaped superior facets and sagittal shaped inferior facets. The lumbar spine, without the rigidity of the rib cage, allows more flexion, extension, and lateral tilt motion, but the sagittal configuration of the facet joints prevent rotation except at the L-5/sacral articulation which usually, again, assumes a more coronal facet configuration.

## 2. Injury Patterns

Mid-thoracic spinal injuries are usually caused by acute flexion rotation axial load forces at the mid-thoracic spine, resulting in either a simple compression fracture of the vertebral body or a complex fracture dislocation in which the vertebral body is fractured and the dorsal elements are also fractured. This allows translation laterally or anteriorly of the upper trunk and upper vertebrae at the fractured segment.

## 3. Injuries at the Thoracolumbar Junction

Most injuries in this area are caused by a combination of flexion, rotation, and axial load. As the chest is rotated and flexed, the rib cage absorbs the flexion energy; the thoracic coronal facets will allow rotation to occur, particularly at the lower thoracic level where the ribs are not attached to the sternum. Therefore, an injury which is centered at T-11/12 will frequently cause a dislocation without fracture of the posterior facets and a slice fracture through the upper portion of the T-12 vertebral body. This injury consists of a fracture of the vertebral body with dislocation of the facet joints.

## 4. Fracture Dislocations of T-12/L-1

If the rotation forces are centered at the T-12/L-1 level, the superior sagittal facets of L-1 block rotation, and the facet on the compression side suffers a fracture which extends down through the superior aspect of the vertebral body of L-1, and the opposite facet, on the distracted side, suffers a dislocation.

If the injury is more axial load with less rotational forces, then the body of L-1 suffers a burst injury in which the hydraulic forces of the more fluid intervertebral disc cause a bursting of the intervertebral body, sending the cortical margins anteriorly, laterally, and posteriorly. The posterior elements of the lamina, spinous processes, and facet joints may be intact or may also be fractured.

## 5. History

When one first sees a patient who has suffered a significant injury to his spine, the details of the accident—whether he was in the automobile or thrown out of the automobile, whether he fell from a height head and shoulders first, or whether he fell from a height feet first, or whether he was restrained in a seatbelt—are important to help diagnose the type of vertebral injury the patient has sustained. External marks on the body, such as bruises over the shoulder or buttocks or fractures of the clavicle, shoulder, os calcis, or pelvis, will also help to pinpoint the area of maximum energy expenditure.

When examining a patient with an injury of the spine, it is important to conduct a systematic general physical examination for other areas of trauma. If the patient has a spinal cord injury, the resultant anesthesia may mask significant and even life-threatening injuries of the abdomen, chest, pelvis, and lower extremities.

## 6. General Evaluation

All patients should be completely disrobed to observe for any areas of bleeding, swelling, or deformity in the spine, extremities, or trunk. Manual palpation of the arms, chest, abdomen, and legs should be conducted for any areas of tenderness or abnormal motion of bones or joints in the lower extremities.

The pattern of breathing should be noted, and the patient should be asked to take a deep breath and to cough. Is he using only his diaphragm for inhalation? Is he also using his intercostals? Does he use his abdominal muscles for forced expiration or coughing? The patient should then be asked for any specific areas of pain or tenderness along the spine. By slipping a hand beneath the patient, the spine can be carefully palpated for any areas of tenderness in the thoracic or lumbar area.

## 7. X-Ray Evaluation

The area of specific interest should be X-rayed before the patient is moved from the original stretcher in the emergency room. A lateral X-ray of any suspected area is taken on a large film. After the X-ray is evaluated for any evidence of fracture, dislocation, or soft tissue swelling, the patient is gently lifted and an A/P X-ray is taken of the suspected area. After these two X-rays of the suspected area are thoroughly evaluated, additional X-rays are taken in the lateral and A/P plane of the rest of the spine and the pelvis to rule out other fractures. An A/P chest X-ray should be taken to observe the soft tissue shadows of the mediastinal viscera to rule out injuries to the aorta and pneumothorax. If the person has paralysis with abdominal anesthesia or if there is any suggestion of intraabdominal pathology, a peritoneal tap and lavage should be performed to rule out intraperitoneal bleeding. If there is no fracture of the pelvis evident on X-ray, an indwelling urethral catheter should be inserted to assess the condition of the urine and monitor urine output. If there is an ileus present, a nasogastric tube should be inserted to maintain decompression of the gastrointestinal tract. A large bore intravenous catheter should be placed in a large vein for administration of necessary fluid or blood. One must be cautious, however, not to over-hydrate a patient who has not had significant blood loss.

## 8. Evaluation of the Cardiovascular Tree

If the patient has a high thoracic spinal cord injury, he may be in a condition of sympathetic spinal shock. This condition occurs when the spinal cord suffers a significant injury in the cervical or upper thoracic area. The cord distal to the level of injury enters a state of areflexia. For a short period of time (up to six to twenty-four hours), the patient will demonstrate a condition of areflexia with hypotonia and a "sympathectomy effect". The vascular tree will dilate, and fluids will accumulate in the peripheral vascular tree. Typically, the patient has a low blood pressure of 90 systolic over 50 or 60 diastolic but does not have a rapid pulse. The pulse averages around 90. The urine output may decrease to 30 cc's per hour. As long as there are no signs of hemorrhage, and the urine output maintains 30 cc's per hour, one should be cautious in administering IV fluids so as not to overload the vascular system. After twenty-four hours, the reflexes begin to recover, and over forty-eight to seventy-two hours the vascular tree begins to contract; there will be diuresis, and, if the patient is overloaded with two or three liters of fluid each day, he may be thrown into pulmonary edema and cardiac failure. Fluids should be carefully monitored, and only fluids which are lost through urinary output, nasogastric suction, and insensible loss, should be replaced during the first three days.

If the patient has a concomitant fractured pelvis, one must be very careful in attempting to insert a urinary catheter. An external urethrogram should be performed by gently inserting the catheter into the penile urethra and injection Renografin dye through the catheter to outline the urethra to assure that there is no rupture of the urethra before inserting the catheter into the bladder. If the catheter meets a resistance at the vesical neck, more Renografin should be inserted through the catheter to ensure that there is no rupture at this junction. After the catheter enters the bladder, a cystogram is performed to document integrity of the bladder.

## 9. Neurological Clinical Evaluation

Documentation of the neurological evaluation depends upon knowledge of the neuro-anatomy of the contents of the spinal canal at each level. There are two anatomical features to remember. The first is that the spinal cord in the adult ends at the inferior aspect of L-1; therefore, the spinal cord segments which are injured do not correspond with the vertebral bony segment level. In the upper thoracic spine, there is only a two to three level difference. The further one descends the thoracic spine, the greater the disparity. For example, the lumbar segments of the spinal cord lie behind the tenth, eleventh, and twelfth vertebral bodies; the sacral segments of the spinal cord (the bladder reflex) are at the vertebral level of T-12/L-1 disc and L-1 body. Therefore, behind any vertebral body in the thoracic spine, there is a segment of spinal cord giving rise to nerve roots which exit several segments lower and also several nerve roots traversing the canal which are also in jeopardy. Injuries to the L-2, L-3, L-4, and L-5 lumbar vertebrae do not cause injuries to the spinal cord. They will cause injuries only to the cauda equina or nerve roots supplying the lumbar and sacral segments of skin and muscle groups.

Injuries at the thoracolumbar junction (T-11/12, T-12/L-1) are the most complex, and the clinical manifestation of these injuries will be discussed in most detail.

## 10. Sensory Evaluation

Sensory evaluation is performed first, since this can be done without moving the patient and can establish a level of suspected paralysis. With the patient lying in the supine position, the pinwheel is first rolled over the face, neck, and arms to establish the patient's response to normal sensation. The pinwheel is then run down over the trunk and onto the upper thighs and legs; any areas of abnormality in patient's response to sharpness are marked. If there is abnormality discovered over the feet or legs or trunk, the pinwheel is brought up from the anesthetic area to the sensate area, and the level is marked, both at the first perception of sensation and at the level of awareness of sharp versus dull. The patient may have a zone of present but abnormal sensation distal to the area of sharp/dull sensation. After this first level is identified, the areas distal to the injury are then examined in more detail to perceive if the patient can feel touch or deep pressure or proprioception of the foot or toes. Response to pinprick and touch over the foot and deep pressure over the Achilles tendon and proprioception of the toes are documented. Two point discrimination has not been found to be as valuable in the foot as it has been in the hand. Two point distance discrimination is very variable in the lower extremities.

After the sensory evaluation, a motor evaluation is conducted—first by asking the patient just to move his toes. The strength of the toe flexors and extensors are determined. The patient is then asked to move his ankles, and the strength is documented. By gently supporting the thigh in the mildly flexed position, the patient can be asked to contract the quadriceps and the hamstrings. This may be quite painful in the face of a fracture of the spine or pelvis. Musles about the hip are difficult to evaluate and cannot be accurately graded in the acute phase; however, one should attempt to elicit a palpable contraction of hip flexors, abductors, adductors, and extensors to verify their presence or absence. The abdominal musles are then evaluated by asking the patient to contract his abdominal musles, as in lifting his head and shoulders isometrically. Note the position and movement of the umbilicus. Active motion of the upper abdominals with paralysis of lower abdominals will cause the umbilicus to move cephalad. Unilateral paralysis of the abdominal will cause the umbilicus to move laterally towards the active side. The intercostal muscles are then observed with deep breathing, and the abdominals are again observed during coughing.

After the gross examination of the sensory and motor evaluation of the lower extremities and trunk, the legs are carefully abducted and the perineal area is examined. The skin around the anus and over the testicles and penis (or labia in the female) is carefully evaluated with a pin to ascertain sharp/dull discrimination on both sides. Also, at this time, the anal wink reflex is observed during pricking of the skin with the pin. A gloved finger is then introduced into the rectum, and the patient is asked to contract the sphincters around the finger to evaluate voluntary sphincter control. During the rectal examination, the perception of deep pressure by the patient can also be documented. The bublocavernosis reflex is then elicited by a quick squeeze of the glans penis, tap on the mons pubis, or a gentle tug on the catheter. If the stimulation causes a reflex contraction of the rectal sphincter, the bulbocavernosus reflex is positive. This indicates that if the patient has a spinal cord injury, it is above the conus and that the patient is not in spinal shock. If the bulbocavernosus and anal wink are negative, and the patient has no sensation or voluntary control, this indicates the injury is either of the conus, the cauda equina, or that the patient is in spinal shock if the injury is above the conus.

## 11. Flaccidity Versus Spasticity

As the patient recovers from spinal shock and the reflexes return, the first reflexes which will be evident will be the perineal reflexes, i.e., the anal wink and the bulbocavernosus. If these are present in the face of complete anesthesia and paralysis, this indicates a complete supra-conal lesion and that the patient is out of spinal shock. The next reflexes which will be seen to recover will be the plantar flexor reflexes of the toe flexor muscles. This is frequently interpreted by the patient as recovering voluntary motor control. However, if the patient can only flex his toes by taking a deep breath, doing a Valsalva maneuver, and straining his upper trunk, then this is most likely a reflex unless he can individually flex the toes of one foot on command without the other foot flexing. The Babinski response is variable and may or may not be present and may be present one day and absent the next day following a severe spinal cord injury. The next and final reflexes to recover are the deep tendon reflexes of the ankle and knee.

Of great importance during the initial evaluation is the cystometrogram. Sophisticated urodynamic studies can be performed which will measure bladder capacity, bladder strength, sphincter control, and detrusor sphincter synergy to help evaluate the magnitude of the injury. A simple cystometrogram can be done by attaching the catheter to a three-way pressure manometer and serially injecting 50 cc aliquots of saline into the bladder and measuring the pressure response on the pressure manometer. Normal bladder sensation and detrusor action will provide a mild contraction and increased pressure with each introduction of 50 cc bolus, but the pressure will gradually go down to base line. As more fluid is injected into the bladder, the resting pressure will slowly rise, and, at about 350 to 400, the patient will get the urge to void, and at 450 or more, the pressure will rise abruptly, and the patient will void around the catheter. If the bladder has suffered a lower motor neuron injury, i.e., a conus or cauda injury, the bladder will be flaccid and fluid will not generate periodic increases in pressure, and the bladder may be filled with 600 to 700 cc's until the elastic limits are met and the pressure rises abruptly without voluntary contraction. If the patient has a spastic bladder, every 50 cc aliquot will result in a high spike of pressure; after 200 to 250 cc's, the pressure will rise precipitously, and involuntary voiding will occur.

This bladder test is particularly of importance in the patient who has a fracture and appears to have no neurological injury. A subtle injury to the conus may produce bladder reflex irregularities with incontinence and loss of erection reflex in the male without other obvious neurological disabilities in the trunk or lower extremities. It is also important on the other end of the scale, in the patient who appears to have a complete paralysis, to document whether the bladder has suffered a lower motor neuron injury with flaccidity or an upper motor neuron injury and develops reflex emptying with spasticity.

## 12. Incomplete Syndromes

If the patient has suffered a fracture of his thoracic spine and has a neurological deficit, but has some sparing of sensation, motor power, or bladder control below the level of injury, it is an "incomplete" or "partial" injury. It is important to ascertain the type and severity of injury to make a prognosis regarding future recovery.

### 13. Brown-Séquard Syndrome

The person who demonstrates weakness of one leg but good ipsilateral sensibility, with decreased sensation and good motor power on the contralateral leg is diagnosed as having a Brown-Séquard syndrome. These patients have a 90% chance of good recovery, both for functional ambulation without aids and control of bowel and bladder.

### 14. Central Cord Syndrome

If the patient has retained sensation to the lower extremities and has sharp/dull discrimination, even though he has a profound or even complete paralysis of the muscles of the lower extremities, he is classified as having a central cord sysndrome, with sparing of the lateral white matter tracts around the periphery of the cord and can be expected to make a significant recovery. Approximately 50% of these patients will recover enough motor power to be ambulatory even though they may have significant spasticity which will hamper their function. Approximately 50% will have recovery of bladder control but will have persistent urinary frequency and urgency.

### 15. Anterior Cord Syndrome

If the patient has only deep pressure perception and proprioception in the lower extremities without sensibility to light touch or sharp/dull discrimination, the patient is placed in the anterior cord syndrome category. With this particular syndrome, it is imperative to examine the perineum. The patient may have sharp/dull pinpoint discrimination around the perineum only, and this would place him in the central cord syndrome, giving him a much better prognosis than the anterior cord syndrome. Only 10% of those with an anterior cord syndrome with deep "protective" sensibility will recover significant functional motor strength in the lower extremities. 30% to 40% of the patients will develop some weak "useless" control of muscles in the feet or legs, but will not be able to use those muscles functionally for ambulation, transfer activities, or wheelchair propulsion.

### 16. Complete Lesions

If the patient has a definite level of anesthesia to all sensibilities and no voluntary muscle control below that level, he is classified as having a complete neurological lesion. The specific, exact level of the lesion is very important to document injury to the cord, conus, or cauda equina in predicting possible recovery.

## 17. Complete Thoracic Paraplegia

Disruptions of the thoracic spine causing complete injuries to the spinal cord virtually always result in complete permanent paraplegia. This spinal cord is tightly enclosed in a narrow canal, and there is no room for mobility, stretching, or impact by bone fracture fragments. The circulation in the mid-thoracic area is also relatively poor compared to the rest of the spinal cord. Therefore, the prognosis for recovery following a severe injury to the mid-thoracic cord which causes immediate complete paraplegia is predicted by the severity of the initial injury. Cord function is not expected to recover, regardless of treatment. Nerve roots traversing the injured spinal canal are more resistant to injury than the spinal cord and may demonstrate progressive recovery for several months following a neuropraxia or axonotmesis type of injury.

## 18. Clinical Findings of Complete Spinal Cord Lesions Secondary to Fractures from T-1 to T-11

Sensation will be at the expected level on the skin dermatome, corresponding to the level of the fracture. The patient may expect to improve one or two levels of skin sensation due to recovery of the nerve roots which are traversing the area of fracture prior to exiting through the neural foramen.

Motor level can be determined by observation and palpation of the intercostal and abdominal muscles. T-9 and T-10 innervate the upper abdominal and T-11 and T-12 innervate the lower abdominal and quadratus lumborum muscles. Reflexes (perineal and deep tendon) may be absent initially but are expected to recover (perineal in six to twenty-four hours, deep tendon up to six weeks).

## 19. Thoracolumbar Junction: Injuries at the T-12/L-1 Level

The spinal cord neural elements at the T-12/L-1 vertebral level consist of the second and third sacral segments of the conus medullaris of the spinal cord. All of the lumbar nerve roots, L-1 through L-5, traverse the spinal canal at this vertebral level prior to exiting through their respective neural foramen more caudally in the vertebral column.

## 20. Root Escape

The spinal cord and conus are more sensitive to injury than the cauda equina nerve roots; therefore, a partial injury may injure the conus medullaris only and spare several or all of the lumbar nerve roots. One must differentiate in the neurologic evaluation, the dermatome segments and muscles innervated by the conus medullaris (spinal cord) and the dermatomes and muscles innervated by the cauda equina (nerve roots). All of the leg muscles and leg skin dermatomes are innervated by the cauda equina. These may be completely absent at the L-1 level and below. Progressive recovery may, however, ensue over the next several months, since the cauda equina may suffer a neurapraxia or even axonotmesis and show progressive recovery. If the conus medullaris suffers a complete injury which persists for twenty-four hours, it reacts like the rest of the spinal cord and will not show progressive recovery. Therefore, the perineal examination (sphincter and perineal skin) will document the cord injury, which, if complete, will be permanent.

A person with a fracture dislocation of T-12 on L-1 may present with no neurological loss whatsoever, or with minor bladder control and erection reflex difficulties only (documented by a cystometrogram), or a more severe conus injury (loss of voluntary bowel and bladder sphincter control, impotence, and incontinence), or a more severe injury which involves the conus and one or more of the lumbar nerve roots. Although a complete conus lesion will not recover, lumbar nerve root injuries may demonstrate progressive recovery. The most severe injury, which would be a complete disruption of all of the lumbar nerve roots as well as the conus medullaris causes a complete T-12 paraplegia, which is permanent.

### 21. Injuries One Level Above the Thoracolumbar Junction: T-11/T-12

These injuries are similar to T-12/L-1 injuries, with two exceptions: 1. This is a supra-conus lesion; therefore, even though the perineal reflexes and sphincter reflexes may be absent initially, they may recover after the person comes out of spinal shock. A patient with this level of injury will be able to develop an automatic reflexly filling/emptying bladder which will kick off on its own after a period of bladder training, whereas the T-12/L-1 injury (which is a conus lesion) disrupts the reflex arch such that the patient will never have an automatic bladder which will fill up and kick off on its own. T-11/T-12 injury will also demonstrate spasticity of the sacrally innervated segments, particularly toe flexors, ankle plantar flexors, and lateral hamstrings. 2. There is much less likelihood of root escape and less chance of progressive cauda equina root recovery.

### 22. Injury One Level Below the Thoracolumbar Junction: L-1/L-2

Injuries of the lumbar spine below L-1 which cause neurological loss are documented by loss of sensation, loss of motor control, loss of bowel and bladder control, and areflexia. These are injuries of the cauda equina distal to the spinal cord. They may demonstrate areas of root escape in which some root segments are functioning and others are not, and they may show progressive root recovery over six weeks to six months as the neurapraxic or axonotmesis lesion of the nerve roots recover.

Frequently, the patient will have retained sensation in the perineum and/or lower extremities but have complete motor paralysis. In this instance, one can usually expect motor recovery to match the neural segments where sensation has been spared. Progressive motor recovery is more common than is sensory recovery. If a person has sensory deficits, these are less likely to show improvement than motor deficits. The ganglion cell of the dorsal sensory nerve root is peripheral to the injury of the nerve in the cauda equina; therefore, while the motor nerve may recover, progressing distally from its motor cell, the sensory nerve has to regenerate proximally up to connections in the spinal cord. This usually does not happen. Neuropraxic lesions may show early progressive recovery of both motor and sensation; however, if the deficit persists for several weeks, only progressive motor recovery can be predicted, and there may be continuing improvement for six to eighteen months.

One cannot accurately predict recovery of injuries to the cauda equina (either at the mid-lumbar level or T-12/L-1 level) as well as one can predict recovery of various spinal cord lesions.

Spasticity only occurs in segments below the level of injury with an intact reflex arc. Therefore, high thoracic spine injuries have great amounts of spasticity ... low thoracic injuries have spasticity only in the sacrally innervated segments ... lumbar injuries which are lower motor neuron injuries do not demonstrate spasticity.

## 23. Thoracolumbar Fractures in Children

Injuries to the thoracolumbar spine may cause injuries to the spinal cord in children. These are more commonly due to being thrown from a bicycle, out of an automobile, or child abuse. Approximately 50% of children who demonstrate spinal cord injuries with paralysis upon physical examination will not demonstrate significant fracture or dislocation of the spinal column on X-ray. The spinal column in a child is so flexible that it may deform enough to injure the spinal cord without actually distrupting. Epiphyseal fracture injuries may cause spinal cord injury and also not be evident on X-ray examination.

Severe injury to the spine in a child may cause a separation of the ring apophysis of the vertebra which may be mildly displaced and not obvious as a fracture on X-ray.

## 24. Quantitative Documentation of Patient Function Following Spinal Cord Injury and Progressive Recovery

Most series documenting spinal cord injuries and recovery use imprecise terms such as "ability to walk" or "functional recovery" as documentation of progressive neurological recovery. The Frankel classification of A, B, C,

D, and E is the most widely used classification to document injury and final recovery states. This is, however, rather grossly subjective when it separates "useless" versus "functional" muscles; it also does not separate "recovery of cord function" versus "cauda equina function". The use of a motor trauma index which documents specific strength of specific musles is an attempt to quantify the amount of muscle paralysis and the amount of functional recovery. Actual specific muscle grading of major groups such as hip flexors, knee extensors, and hamstrings is difficult in the acute stage, but an approximate assessment of their function on a numerical scale has improved the ability to more accurately document neurological recovery following an injury and specifically following various modes of treatment.

## 25. Summary

When faced with a patient with a fracture of the spine and possible injury to the neural contents, one must carefully evaluate other organ systems for any evidence of multiple injuries and accurately document the neurological assessment and correlate the neurological assessment with the radiographic level of injury. Only with an accurate initial assessment can we rationally select appropriate treatment modalities and evaluate the outcome of different treatment regimens.

### References


1. Bosch A, Stauffer ES, Nickel VL (1971) Incomplete traumatic quadriplegia: a ten year review. J Am Med Assoc 216: 473–478
2. Kaufer H (1984) The thoracolumbar spine. In: Rockwood and Green (eds) Fractures. J. B. Lippincott Company, Philadelphia, pp 1036–1092
3. Stauffer ES (1982) Rehabilitation of the spinal cord injured patients. In: Rothman and Simeone (eds) Spine. W. B. Saunders Company, Philadelphia, Chapter 19, pp 1118–1131

# Radiological Investigations

H. Hacker

Department of Neuroradiology, J. W. Goethe University, Frankfurt
(Federal Republic of Germany)

With 5 Figures

## Contents



## 1. Radiological Investigations

The patient with suspected vertebral trauma should have a radiological examination immediately to prevent possible further displacement of fragments. Until the radiological work-up is finished and a fracture has been ruled out, the patient is treated as having spinal trauma. If neurological symptoms and signs suggest involvement of the spinal cord or cauda equina, the case is considered to be a radiological emergency.

The transport to the X-ray table has to be done with the greatest of care to avoid any passive bending. If three persons to carry the patient are not available, a board or a strong plastic sheet with handles is helpful. A plastic sheet is transparent to X-rays and the patient may lie on this until all examinations are completed.

## 2. Methods of Investigation

At the present time neuroradiological method are undergoing rapid change. Computerised tomography has become a universally available technique, magnetic resonance imaging will in a few years be the standard examination for the content of the spinal canal and will replace many myelographies. There is however a drawback for all tomographic methods, which for ideal results require the spine to be oriented in a straight line. Even a pathological curvature of the spine is no problem for examinations in the sagittal plane as practiced with conventional tomography and MRI. Additional lateral scoliosis may prevent successful tomography. The situation is worse for the axial technique of CT. Here the examination plane has to be oriented for any given area perpendicular to the spinal canal. Otherwise errors in reading the images may occur and no reliable judgement of the content of the spinal canal is possible. For this reason any radiological examination of the spine should start with plain X-rays or at least a digital survey radiograph taken in the CT-scanner (scout-view, scanogram, topogram) in both lateral and A.P. projections. Displacements and contortions will thus be diagnosed and corrections for tomography may be done. Also most fractures of the vertebral bodies may be so diagnosed. If the trauma involves two or three vertebrae only we like to obtain a high detail film by coning down or by the use of a Vienna tube. Especially in the lumbar region, oblique views for the pedicles and facet joints will show luxations and fractures of the arch and joints.

For further detail or if a fracture is only suspected, conventional tomography is still helpful, especially for the vertebral body. Small central infractions by the nucleus may only be seen by tomography. The arch and articulations however are best demonstrated by axial CT.

In severe and clearly localized trauma the neuroradiological examination may be started immediately on the CT-scanner using digital radiography for survey before proceeding to axial scans. Secondary to plain films CT is always necessary if signs of involvement of nervous structures are present. CT is also mandatory if fractures of the posterior part of the vertebral body or the arch are suspected. It is of importance to rule out any displacement of bone fragments into the spinal canal.

The spinal cord itself can only be seen clearly if a sufficient large subarachnoid space around it is present. As a rule this is rare and it cannot be expected if there is swelling of the cord. Blood will be seen only if a localized hematoma is present. The density of blood is only rarely as high as in an intracerebral hemorrhage. Blood therefore may be easily overlooked. Due to the relatively large content of csf, diagnosis of the spinal canal and the nerves is easier below the conus. Intrathecal iodine contrast will help to outline the spinal cord and the nerves clearly. The necessary spinal tap will also give information regarding blood in the subarachnoid space. If the condition of the patient permits conventional myelography with water-soluble contrast will be done first, followed by CT. Since the introduction of Metrizamid more non-ionic iodinated substances have come into use. In our department Solutrast 250 M (Byk-Gulden), 6–10 ml, has been used without side effects.

As the medulla can mostly not be seen properly without contrast, MRI will in future become the method for early detection of any medullary trauma. However this technique must first be available in all hospitals where there is neurosurgery, and second echo-sequences for short examination times must be developed. Also special spinal coils should be used. The advantage of seeing the spinal cord in excellent quality over several segments, the ease of seeing displacements, compression or hematomas will make this the most important examination. It gives the most specific information and allows objective therapeutic decisions. CT will then be a secondary technique for better definitions of subtle bony changes.

However at present CT is the generally available technique. A few technical notes must be given: The examination has always to be conducted in a way for the best visualisation of bone and of soft tissue. This affords that each set of raw-data has to be calculated twice. Using only the large bone window may sometimes be adequate, but lacks all the fine information for bone. For reformation in other planes the slice thickness should be 4 mm or less either overlapping or contiguous. Movements of the patient between two scans should be noted, because it results in a false step when reformatting is done, this may mimick displacement of vertebrae. In later controls that method will be used which previously showed the lesion best.

## 3. Diagnostic Findings

Radiology in trauma is always an incomplete description of lesions as a late result of some momentarily very strong displacements, tensions, compressions, and shearing movements. Immediately following the impact there is a relative realignment by the elasticity of bones, ligaments, muscles, and of other tissue.

Even with all the new imaging tools we will only see part of the actual traumatic lesions as the topical order is restored to a great extent. Bearing this in mind, we may proceed to a descriptive listing of the main findings.

Trauma most frequently involves the lower thoracic and the upper lumbar spine. Compression of one or more vertebral bodies involving the ventral and upper part with a decrease in height, often only ventrally, is the common finding. A similar deformation of vertebral bodies is frequent in the kyphotic middle thoracic spine in the elderly or osteoporotic patient. With the axial cuts in CT we have learned—as have others—that in a flattened vertebra of traumatic origin a fracture line in the spongiosa is often seen (Fig. 1). The infraction of a nucleus pulposus into the spongiosa is best seen in conventional tomograms in the sagittal plane (Fig. 2).

The severity of fractures is scaled from slight ventral depression to an

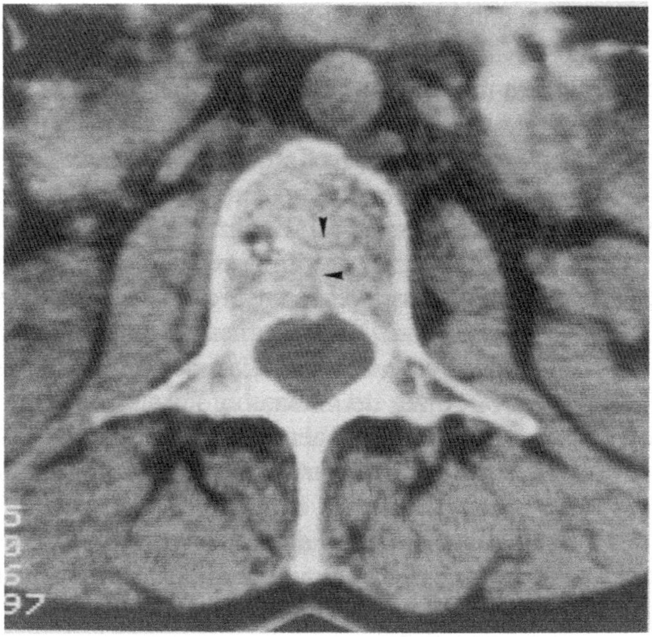

Fig. 1. Small irregular lines in the spongiosa of a fractured vertebra—prooven on adjacent slices. Similar lines, more straight and even, in the center of a vertebral body arranged in a Y-form pattern may correspond to normal vascular channels. Beware of wrong diagnosis!

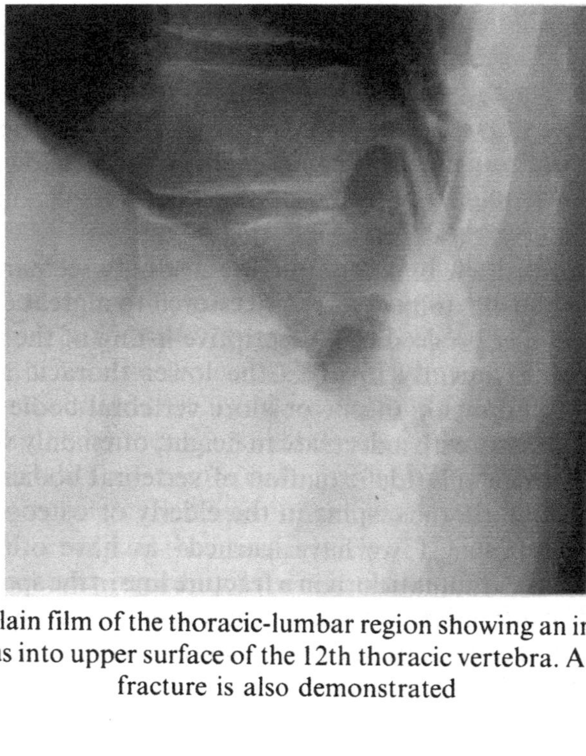

Fig. 2. Lateral plain film of the thoracic-lumbar region showing an infarction of the nucleus pulposus into upper surface of the 12th thoracic vertebra. A slight wedging fracture is also demonstrated

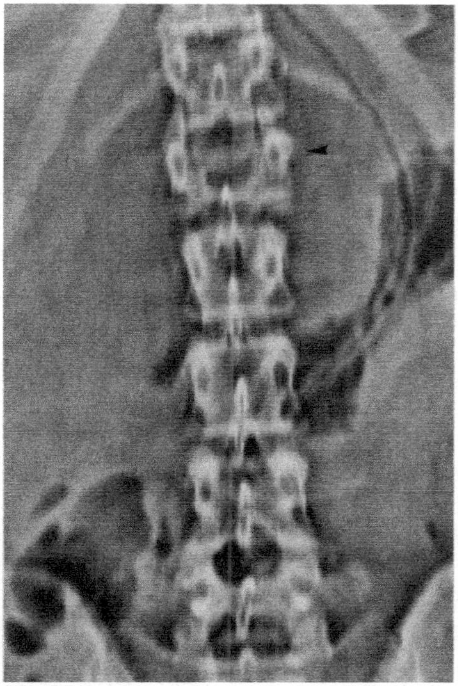

Fig. 3a. a.p. digital roentgenogram (topogram) demonstrates the interest of this technique. The pedicles of the first lumbar vertebra have a greater distance than those above or below. Signs of a dorsal bursting fracture of this vertebra with fracture of the arch

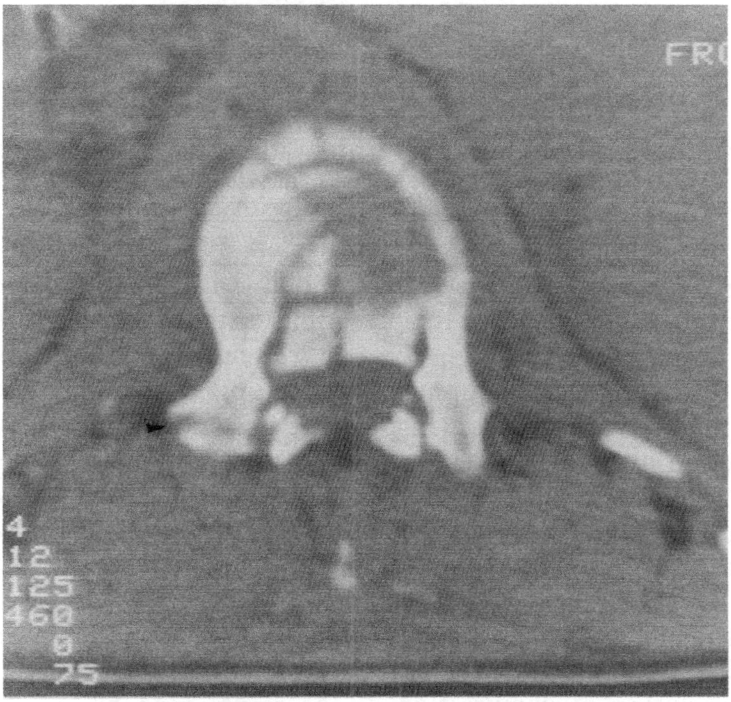


Fig. 3b. Same patient. Axial cut of L 1, demonstrating the bursting. Displacement of bone fragments into the spinal canal, fracture of the articular process

actual bursting of the vertebral body with fragments being pushed into the spinal canal ventral, lateral and sometimes dorsal. The spinal canal may then be narrowed. Some millimeters upward from such a bursting fracture the axial cut through the next vertebra shows a normal vertebra with a surrounding wreath of bone fragments, when a healthy vertebra is pushed into the fractured one (Fig. 3b).

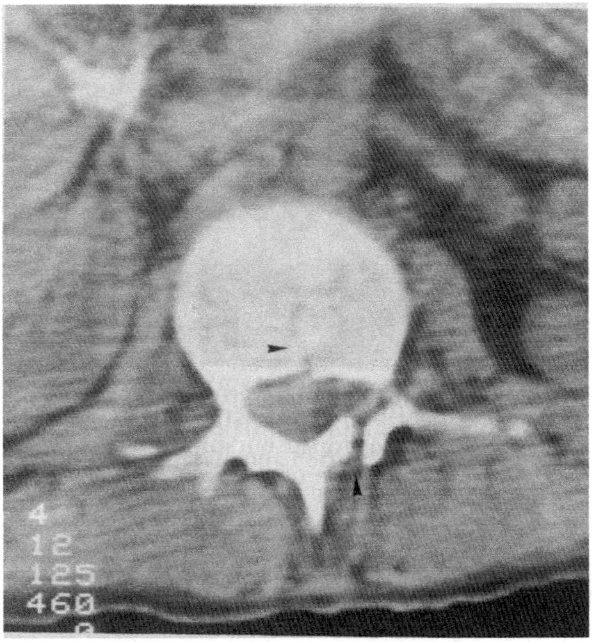


Fig. 4. Fracture of vertebral body and the arch with displacement and deformation of the spinal canal

A horizontal fracture of one vertebral body with lateral deplacement is rare, but will be diagnosed on the plain films or the scout-view. Lateral or anterior-posterior displacement of one vertebral body on the others signifies fracture of the arch or articular facets often followed by dislodgement of an intervertebral disc (Fig. 4). The posterior part of the vertebra may fracture at many points. In the lumbar spine oblique projections disclose fractures of the pedicles or facets. CT has the advantage of demonstrating the whole posterior part of the vertebrae at once, thus giving more complete information. Also disalignment will be seen as can the soft tissue in the intervertebral foramen.

The spinal canal deserves most attention. Even small bone fragments may press on the spinal cord (Figs. 5a, b).

The exclusion of compression of the spinal cord by soft tissue or hematoma is often possible only after the application of intrathecal contrast. In severe trauma with swelling of the cord only a complete block for contrast can be diagnosed by myelography and CT. Probably MRI

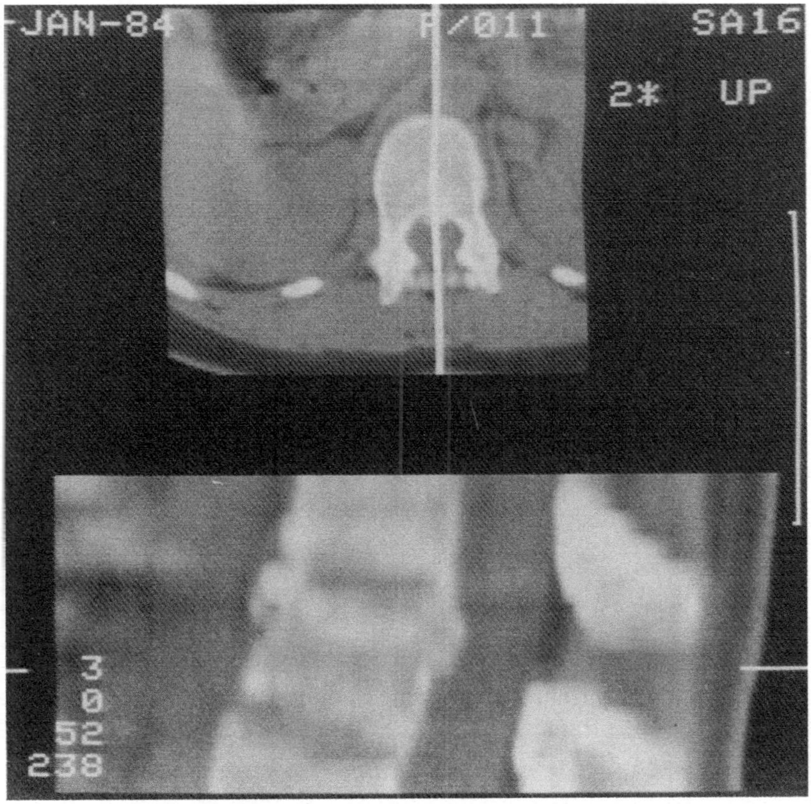


Fig. 5a. Reformatting of a fracture involving the upper surface of the first lumbar vertebra. The displacement of material from bone and intervertebral disc is best seen in the lateral reformatting, which discloses considerable narrowing of the spinal canal

could help to differentiate the cause of a block for contrast, thus proceeding the possibility of planning operative interventions more precisely.

Nerve root avulsions as may be seen in the cervical spine are rare in the lumbar region. This as well as a dural tears will be shown by the leak of contrast in myelography or in CT.

A negative first examination does not rule out thoracic or lumbar vertebral fracture. Brocher stresses the fact that fractures may be seen only after 8 weeks or later. However they are generally partial ventral lesions of the vertebral body. However the patient's complaints of back pain weeks after an accident should prompt late X-ray control. Such delayed fractures are more common in older patients or in osteoporotic vertebrae.

Another late diagnosis now being diagnosed with increased frequency is the finding of intramedullary cystic lesions which are presumed to have followed spinal contusion. This will only be seen in MRI.

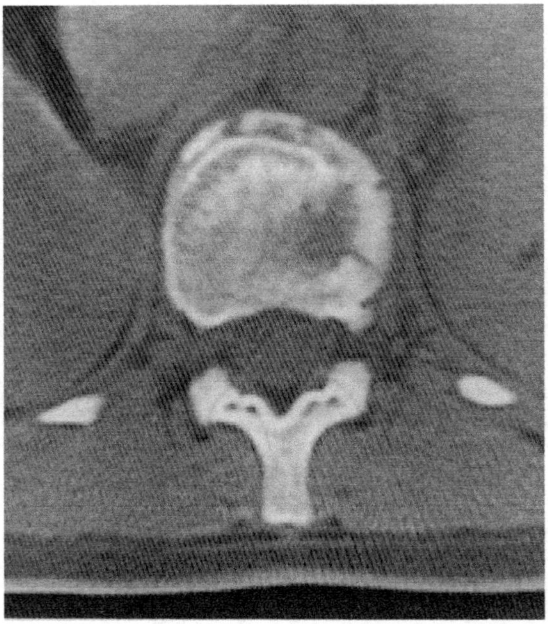

Fig. 5b. 12th thoracic vertebra of the same patient, cut near to the intervertebral space. A wreath of bone fragments from the 1st lumbar vertebra is surrounding the healthy one

The pathology of traumatic changes in the spinal canal and the spinal cord will be known to us only when more observations with MRI are available. It can be expected that this will give a new understanding of neurological symptoms after a thoracic spine trauma, which may not present bony changes.

## 4. How to Do It

Fracture of vertebral body suspected:
— plain films in lateral and a.p. projection;
— lumbar region: additional oblique views;
— tomography in sagittal plane to rule out infraction of upper surface.

Severe bony lesion and suspected fractures of neural arch:
— plain films;
— CT.

Signs of involvement of nervous system:

a) no immediate danger to cord:

— plain films;
— CT;
— MRI (if possible);
— evtl. myelography and myelo-CT;

b) cord or cauda involved (Emergency—Immediate examination!):

— CT *with* scout view in two planes;
— MRI (if possible);
— evtl. myelography and myelo-CT.

## References

1. Brant-Zawadzki M, Jeffrey RB Jr, Minagi H, Pitts LH (1982) High resolution CT of thoracolumbar fractures. Am J Roentgenol 138: 699 – 705 and AJNR 3: 69 – 74
2. Brocher JEW (1962) Die Wirbelsäule und ihre Differentialdiagnose. Thieme, Stuttgart
3. Calenoff L (1981) Radiology of spinal cord injury. Year Book Medical Publishers, London
4. Epstein BS (1976) The spine: a radiological text and atlas. Lea and Febiger, Philadelphia
5. Faerber EN, Wolpert SM, Scott RM, Belkin SC, Carter L (1979) Computed tomography of spinal fractures. J Comput Assist Tomogr 3: 657 – 661
6. Gehweiler JA, Daffner RH, Osborne RL (1981) Relevant signs of stable and unstable thoracolumbar vertebral column trauma. Skeletal Radiol 7: 179 – 183
7. Gehweiler JA, Osborne RL, Becker RF (1980) The radiology of vertebral trauma. W. B. Saunders, New York
8. Griffiths ET, McCormick CC (1981) Post-traumatic syringomyelia (cystic myelopathy). Paraplegia 19: 81 – 88
9. Haughton VM (1983) Computed tomography of the spine. Churchill Livingstone, London
10. Laasonen EM (1977) Myelography for severe thoracolumbar injuries. Neuroradiology 13: 165
11. McAfee C, Yuan A, Frederickson BE, Lubicky P (1983) The value computed tomography in thoracolumbar fractures. An analysis of one hundred consecutive cases and a new classification. JBJS 64A: 461 – 473
12. Newton HT, Potts G (1983) CT of the spine and spinal cord. Clavadel Press, San Francisco
13. Pettersson H, Harwood-Nash DCF (1982) CT and myelography of the spine and cord. Springer, Berlin Heidelberg New York
14. Shuman WP, Rogers JV, Sickler ME, Hanson JA, Crutcher JP, King HA, Mack LA (1985) Thoracolumbar burst fractures: CT dimensions of the spinal canal relative to postsurgical improvement. Am J Neuroradiol (Baltimore) 6: 337 – 341
15. Vervon JD, Silver JR, Olry A (1982) Post-traumatic syringomyelia. Paraplegia 20: 339 – 364

# Intraoperative Ultrasound in Neurotraumatology: Brain, Spinal Cord and Cauda equina

G. J. Dohrmann

Section of Neurosurgery, University of Chicago Medical Center, Chicago, Illinois (U.S.A.)

and

J. M. Rubin

Department of Radiology, University of Michigan Hospitals, Ann Arbor, Michigan (U.S.A.)

With 10 Figures

**Contents**



## I. Introduction

Recently, real-time ultrasound imaging has been developed for use in the neurosurgical operating room to allow the neurosurgeon to "explore" the brain or spinal cord/cauda equina without opening the dura[1–10]. The major applications for ultrasound imaging intraoperatively have been in patients with tumors, cysts or abscesses; ultrasound has been used for localization,

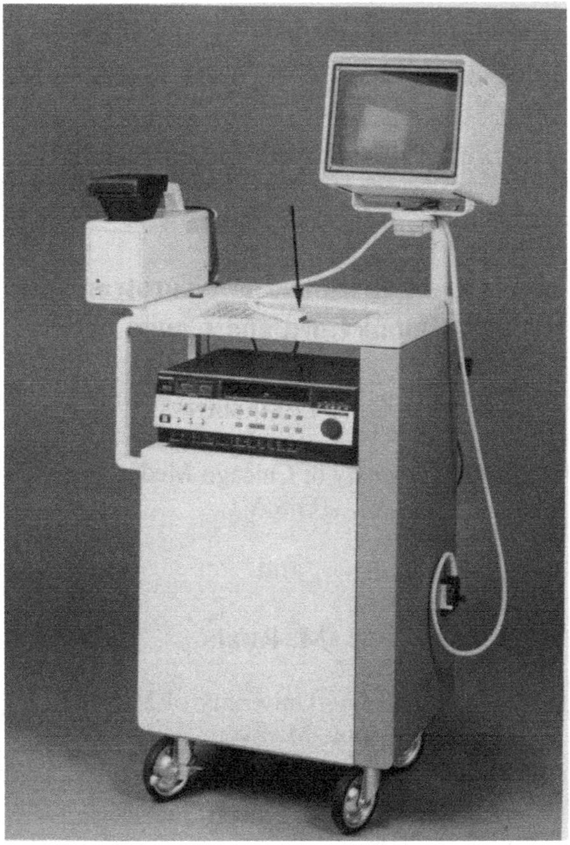

Fig. 1. Real-time ultrasound scanner designed for intraoperative use. Scanhead (arrow) is resting atop the pressure-sensitive control panel; videorecorder is seen below. Polaroid camera is attached to scanner on left; videoscreen is on right. (Codman and Shurtleff, Inc., Randolph, MA 02368, U.S.A.)

characterization and instrumentation of these lesions[3–5, 7, 9]. In neurotrauma, ultrasound can also be of help to the neurosurgeon in localizing intracerebral hematomas as well as indriven bone fragments or foreign bodies (including radiolucent glass and plastic). The purpose of this chapter is to describe the technique of intraoperative ultrasound scanning in the operating room and to illustrate its utility in patients with traumatic lesions involving brain or spinal cord/cauda equina.

## II. The Ultrasound Scanner

An ultrasound scanner (Figs. 1 and 2) consists of a control panel, a videoscreen, a videorecorder and a scanhead that is connected to the scanner by a cable. Ultrasound is produced by transducers within the

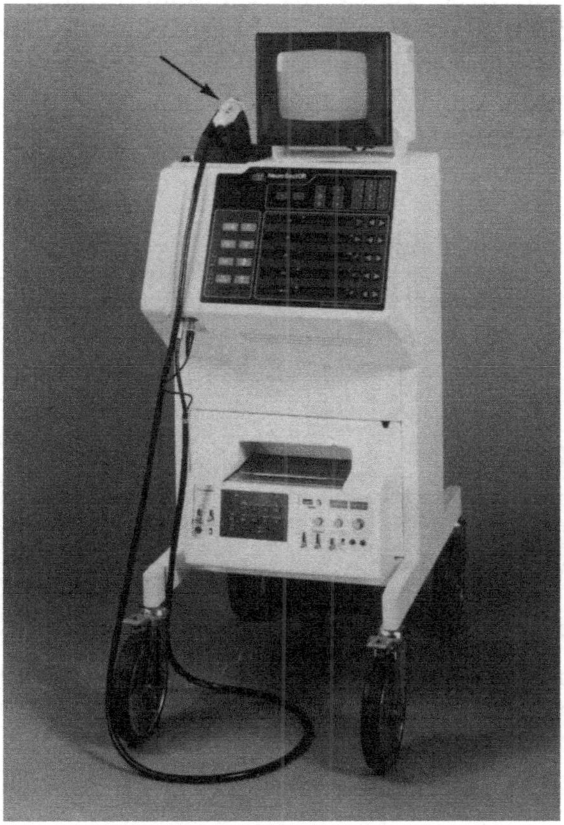

Fig. 2. Another real-time ultrasound scanner designed for intraoperative use. Scanhead (arrow) is connected to scanner by cable. Pressure-sensitive control panel is seen in the center of the scanner with the videoscreen above and the videorecorder below. (Advanced Technology Laboratories, Inc., Bellevue, WA 98005, U.S.A.)

scanhead (Fig. 3). The ultrasound waves travel into the central nervous system tissue and the ultrasound waves echoing back are analyzed by a computer within the scanner. This digital information is displayed as a gray scale on the videoscreen of the scanner. The more echogenic the tissue, the more white it appears (such as tumors or hemorrhage), and less echogenic areas (such as cerebrospinal fluid) are seen as black; the brain is displayed as shades of gray. Multiple images are produced per second and, therefore, physiological motion can be seen. Because of the dynamic aspects of this technique, it is termed "real-time" imaging. If most ultrasound waves are reflected back from an object (such as bone, glass or metal fragments), the object will appear on the videoscreen as very white with "shadowing" behind it, because the ultrasound waves have not passed through it. Instruments, if kept within the width of the scan plane, can be seen and instrumentation may be guided by continuous ultrasound imaging. Transducers of different frequencies can be used as needed: lower frequency transducers (3 mHz) give greater penetration but less resolution than those of higher frequency (5 and 7.5 mHz) that give greater resolution but do not penetrate as deeply into the tissue.

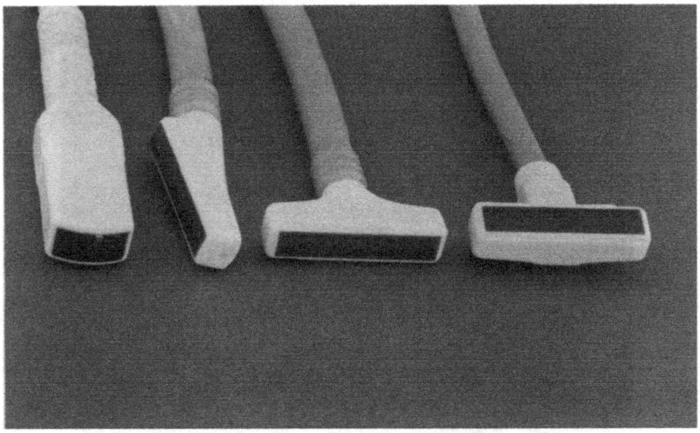

Fig. 3. Ultrasound scanheads for intraoperative imaging. (Note the various sizes and shapes for use depending upon the structure being imaged and the type of operative exposure)

## III. Intraoperative Technique[3]

The control section of ultrasound scanners, specifically designed for intraoperative use (Codman and ATL scanners) are pressure sensitive panels. As such, a sterile transparent plastic drape can be used to cover this panel so that the neurosurgeon may control it by touching the appropriate parts of it during the operation. Quality of image as well as size of image may be adjusted via this control panel. For intraoperative use, the scanhead is covered by a sterile plastic drape. Acoustic coupling is assured by the application of acoustic gel to the surface of the scanhead prior to placement of the plastic bag over it.

For imaging of brain, the sterilely-draped scanhead is then placed on the surface of dura or the exposed cortex (Fig. 4). Several drops of saline are used for acoustic coupling. The brain beneath the scanhead is then imaged dynamically on the videoscreen. The orientation of the scanhead determines the scan plan obtained. If the scanning is done from a lateral direction, the scanhead may be held to provide a coronal section or turned 90° to give a transaxial section. If the craniectomy/craniotomy is near the vertex, the brain may be imaged sagittally or coronally.

For imaging of the contents of the spinal canal, the patient is placed on the operating table in the prone position[2]. After laminectomy (ultrasound is greatly attenuated by bone), the wound is filled with saline. The sterilely-draped scanhead is then applied to the saline and the spinal cord, and associated structures are then imaged on the videoscreen. Longitudinal or

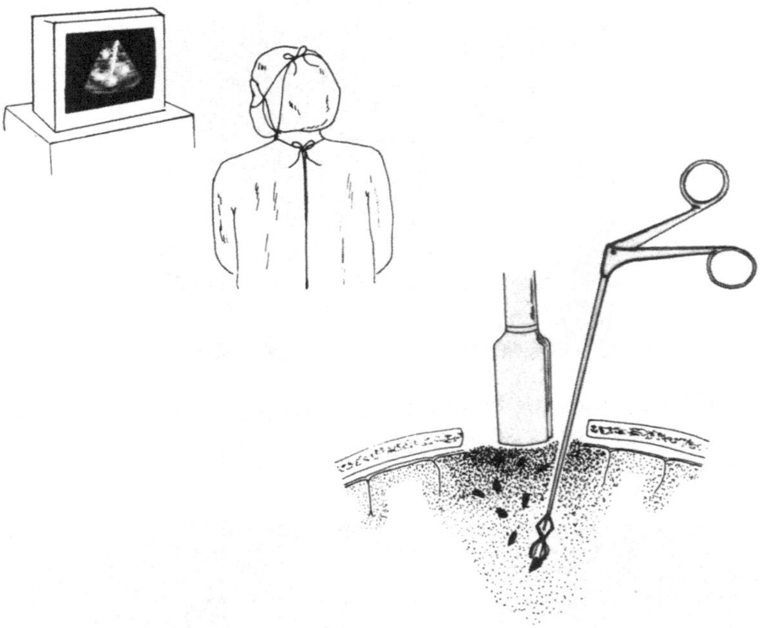

Fig. 4. Line drawing showing use of real-time ultrasound imaging in a patient with a penetrating head injury. Indriven bone fragments, as shown here, or foreign bodies can be identified and removed using this dynamic intraoperative imaging

cross-sections of spinal cord can be obtained depending upon how the ultrasound scan plane is orientated.

Dynamic imaging of the brain or spinal cord may be recorded on videotape using the recorder built into the ultrasound scanner.

## IV. Traumatic Lesions of Brain

Usually the localization of intracranial hematomas presents no problem to the neurosurgeon. Hematomas often occur over the surface of the brain or occur within the brain but present in the operating room as eroding through the cortical surface. Sometimes there is hematoma formation within a contused portion of brain that is not apparent on the computed

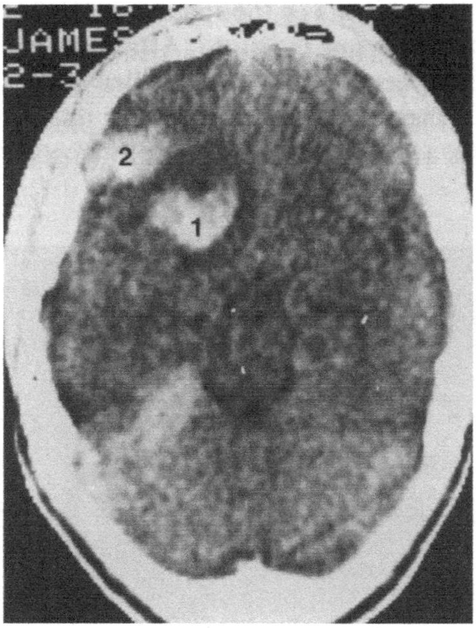


Fig. 5A. CT scan showing two hematomas (*1* and *2*) in the left frontal lobe

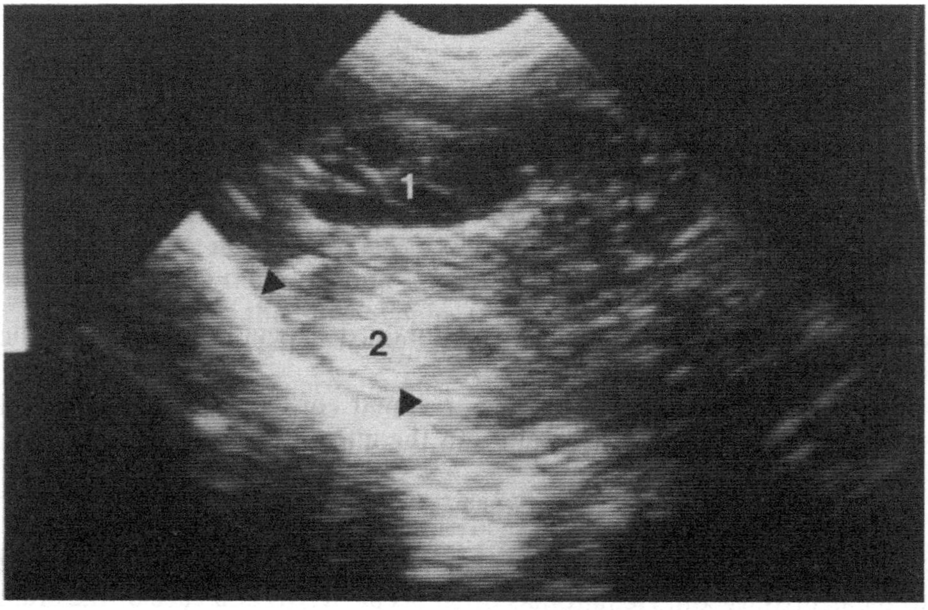


Fig. 5B. Sagittal ultrasound scan showing the two hematomas—one hematoma is less echogenic (*1*) and the other is more echogenic (*2*); floor of anterior fossa (large arrowheads)

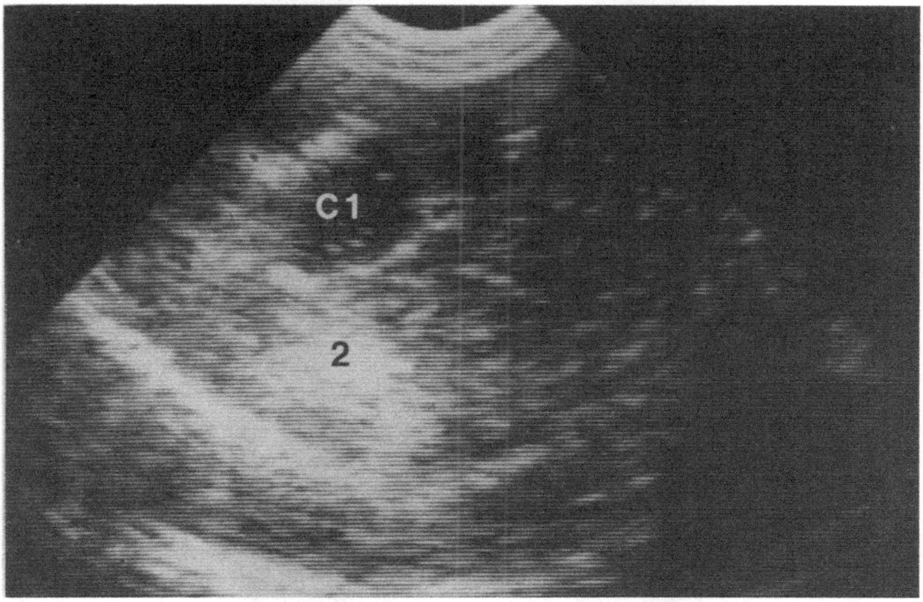


Fig. 5C. Evacuation of the more superficial hematoma, hematoma #1; however, the neurosurgeon thought that both hematomas had been evacuated. The wound was filled with saline and ultrasound imaging showed that the deeper hematoma (*2*) had not been evacuated. Saline within cavitiy of superficial hematoma (*C1*). (Note that echogenic dots within the saline are air bubbles)

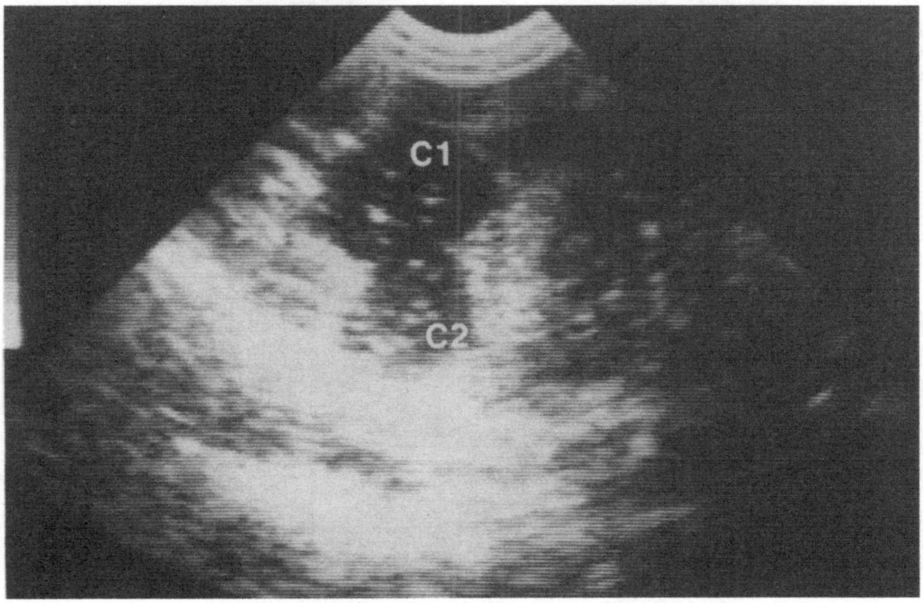


Fig. 5D. Evacuation of deeper hematoma, hematoma #2 as well; wound filled with saline and cavities of both hematomas (*C1* and *C2*) can be seen. (Note echogenic air bubbles within the saline)

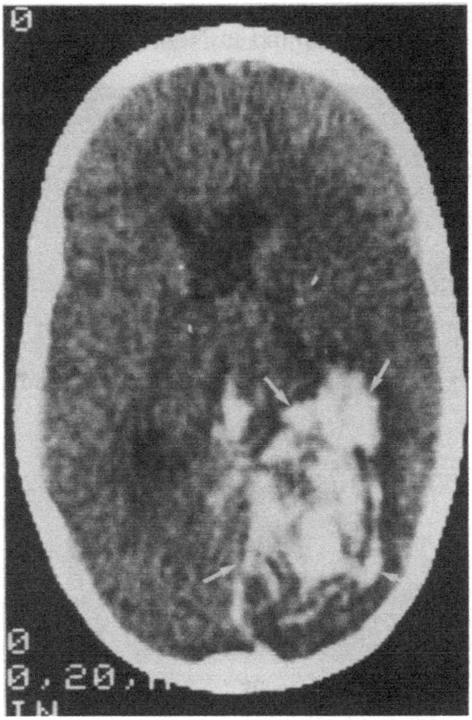

Fig. 6A. CT scan of patient with what appears to be hematoma (arrows) filling most of the posterior portion of the right cerebral hemisphere

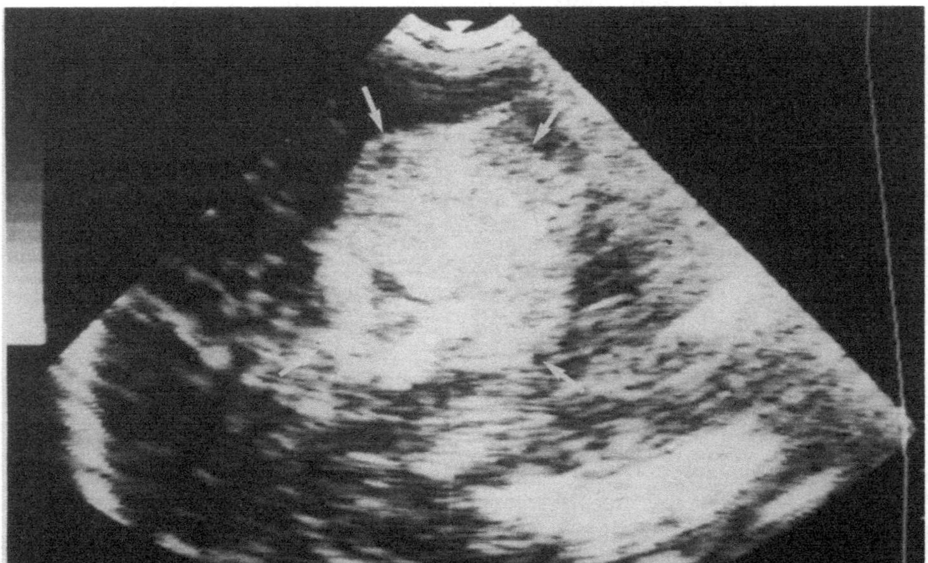

Fig. 6B. Intraoperative ultrasound scan showing that the main mass, the hematoma (arrows), is actually much smaller than it appeared on CT scan. This hematoma was evacuated and most of the posterior cerebral hemisphere was spared; the patient did well

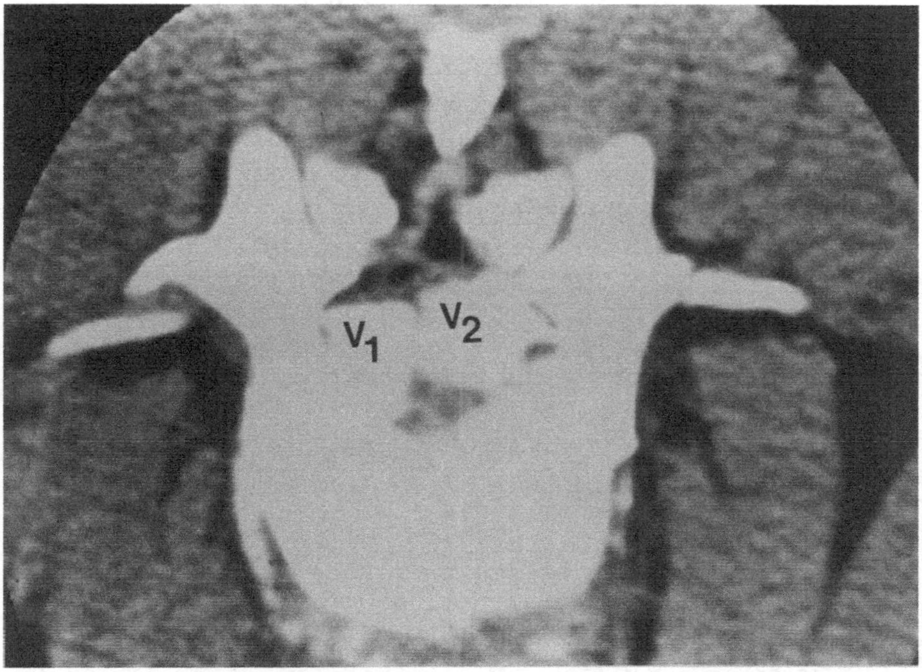


Fig. 7A. CT scan in a patient with a spine fracture and bone fragments (*V1* and *V2*) impinging on the spinal cord

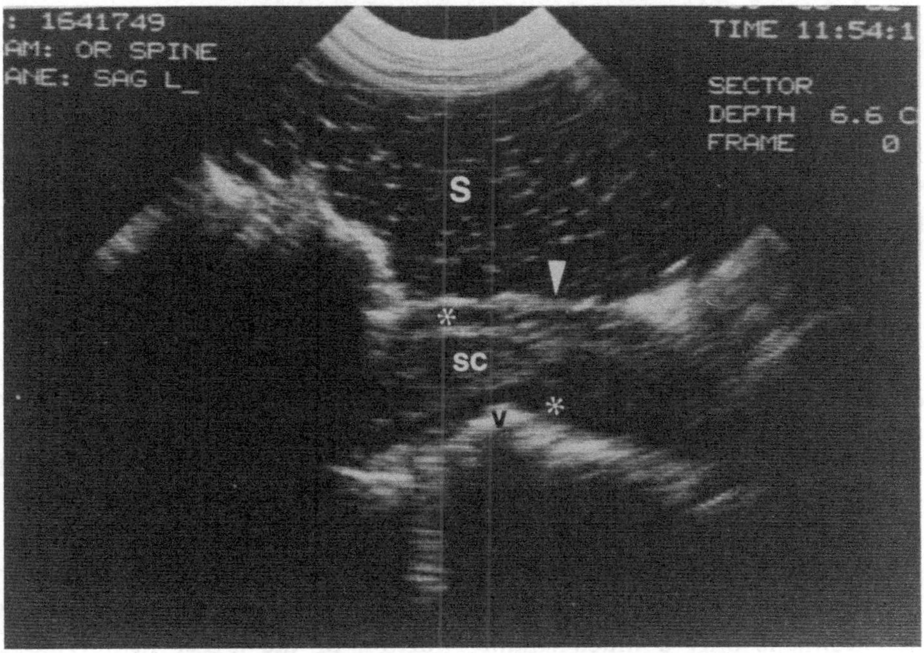


Fig. 7B. Longitudinal ultrasound scan following laminectomy showing the posterior dura (arrowhead), spinal cord (*SC*), subarachnoid space (asterisks) and posteriorly displaced bone fragment from vertebral body (*V*). (Note echogenic air bubbles in the saline (*S*) used to fill the wound to do the ultrasound imaging)

tomographic (CT) scan because the CT scan was taken sometime prior to the operation and hemorrhage can occur into contused brain at varying intervals following trauma. Intraoperative ultrasound can identify all areas of intracerebral hemorrhage, and the neurosurgeon may then plan the most safe and precise way of evacuating them.

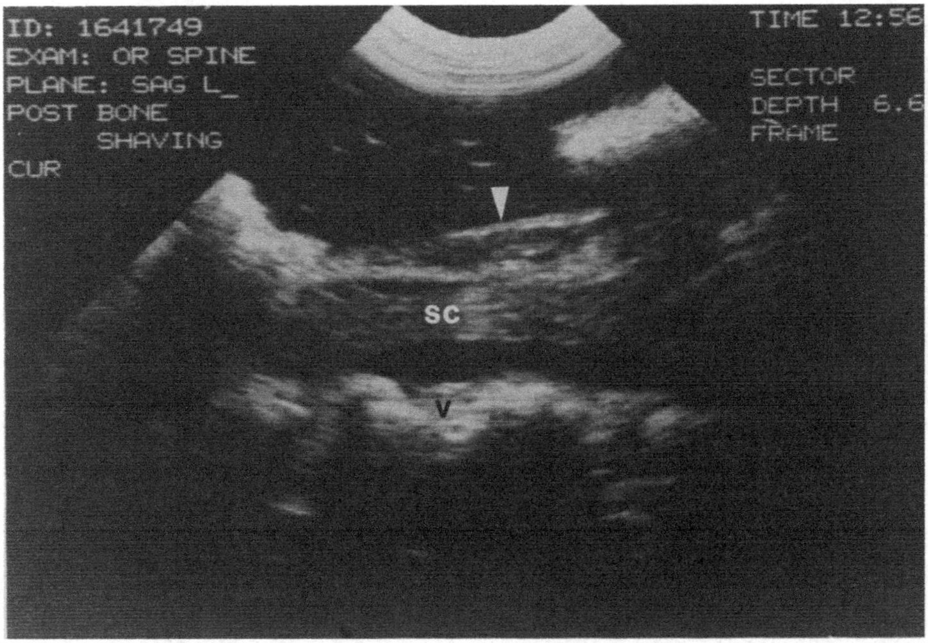


Fig. 7C. Longitudinal ultrasound scan following placement of rods to straighten spine. Note how bone fragment from vertebral body (*V*) has "snapped back" into position and that the spinal cord (*SC*) can be seen to be decompressed. (Note: Blood has layered on posterior dura making it appear thicker [arrowhead] than in Fig. 7B.) (Figs. 7A, B, and C courtesy of Dr. B. A. Green, U.S.A.)

If several adjacent hematomas are noted, ultrasound can be used to check that they were all evacuated. The wound is filled with saline and ultrasound imaging done. Occasionally one of the hematomas might have been missed and that would then be identified and evacuated (Figs. 5A, B, C, and D).

Sometimes on the CT scan there is a mass effect from a hematoma that appears to fill much of one of the lobes of the cerebral hemisphere; however, with ultrasound imaging it can sometimes be demonstrated that a solid hematoma is only a much smaller portion of the larger hemorrhagic-appearing area (Figs. 6A and B). In that case, a topectomy may be performed over the main portion of the hematoma, and the hematoma could be evacuated. The remainder of the "large hematoma" seen on the CT

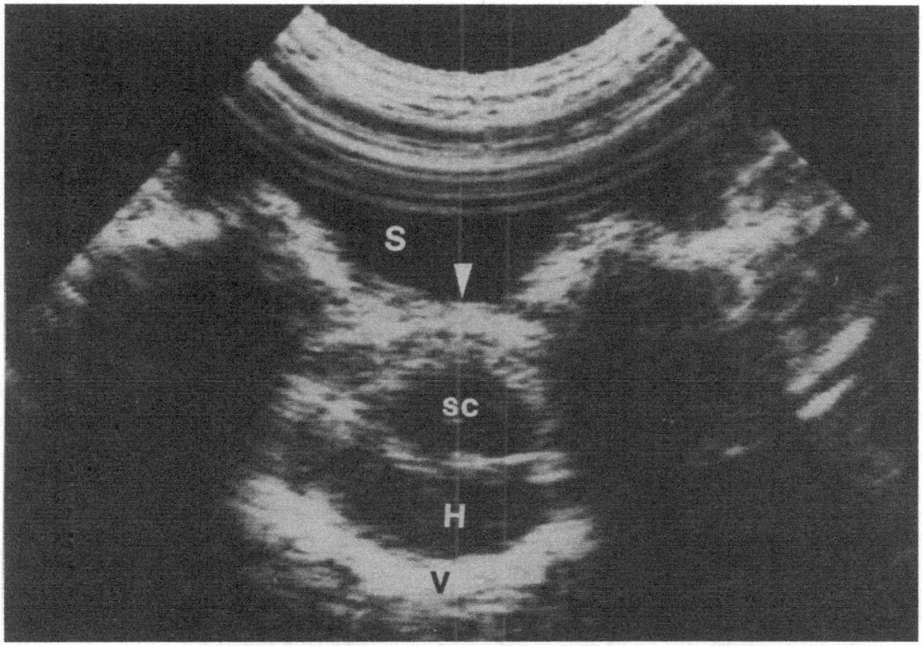


Fig. 8A. Cross-sectional intraoperative ultrasound scan in a patient with spine trauma and a hematoma (*H*) anterior to the spinal cord (*SC*) displacing the spinal cord posteriorly. Posterior surface of dura with some blood layered on it (arrowhead); saline filling wound (*S*); vertebral body (*V*)

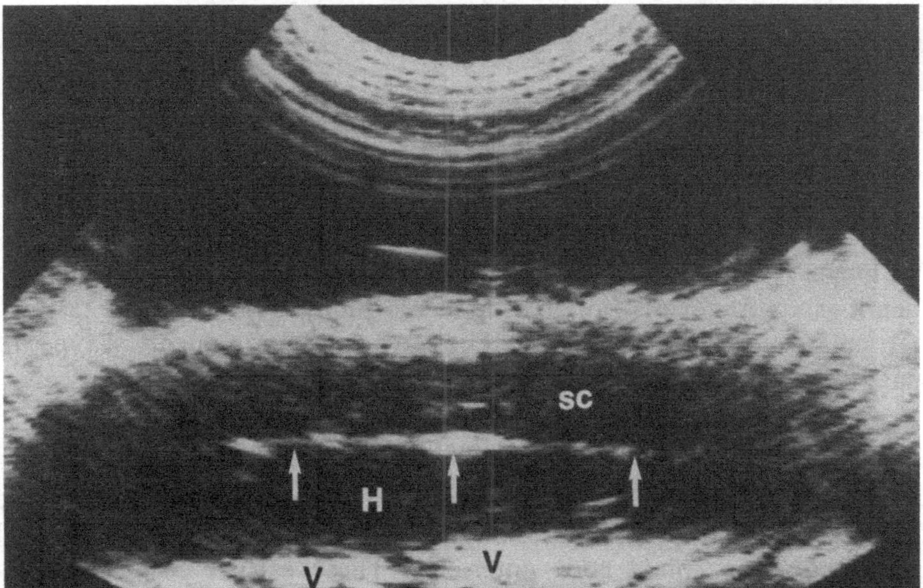


Fig. 8B. Longitudinal ultrasound scan in same patient. Spinal cord (*SC*); anterior surface of spinal cord (arrows); hematoma (*H*); vertebral bodies (*Vs*)

scan was accounted for by tracking of blood into the tissues. For this reason, much of the lobe could be saved as the main mass was removed.

In penetrating injuries of the brain, the main goals are to debride the brain and treat mass effect if present. Ultrasound can image a bullet tract within the brain and also the fragments of bone or bullet fragments. As such, the indriven fragments can be identified and removed easily (Fig. 4).

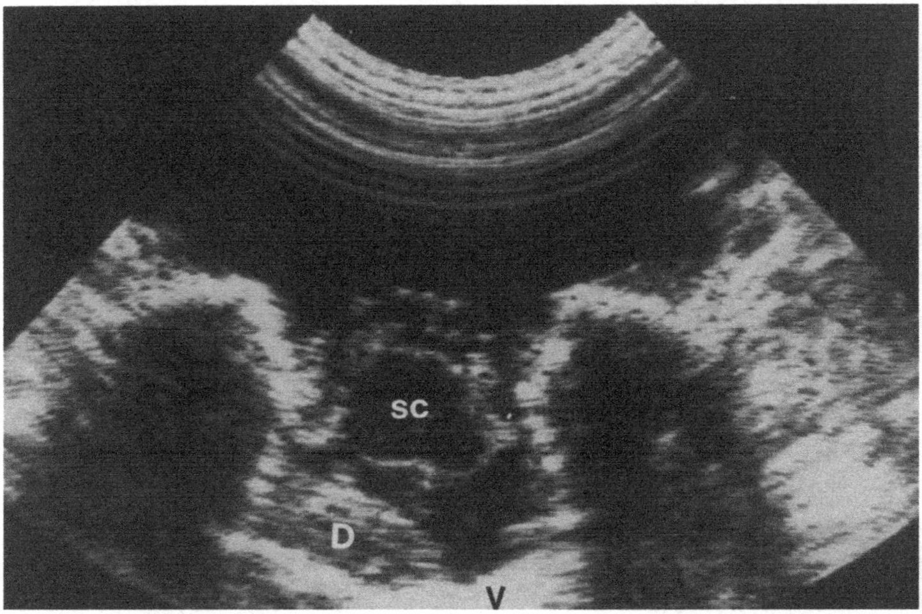


Fig. 9. Cross-sectional intraoperative ultrasound scan in patient with herniation of thoracic disc (*D*) post-trauma. Spinal cord (*SC*); vertebral body (*V*)

No longer is it necessary to use X-ray in the operating room to attempt to identify such fragments—often a time-consuming and frustrating task. In particular, such radiolucent foreign bodies as plastic fragments or types of glass fragments can be visualized with ultrasound.

## V. Trauma to the Spinal Cord/Cauda equina

Spinal cord trauma is often associated with spine fractures. Bone fragments from the vertebral body may be displaced posteriorly and impinge on the spinal cord anteriorly. These can be identified with ultrasound imaging and be removed or they may be seen to "snap back" into position after the placement of rods to straighten and stabilize the spine (Figs. 7A, B, and C). Hematomas anterior to the spinal cord can be visualized (Figs. 8A and B) as well as those located within the spinal cord itself.

In trauma, central disc herniation and the degree of spinal cord compression may be seen intraoperatively using ultrasound (Fig. 9). After excision of the disc and/or fragments of disc material within the spinal

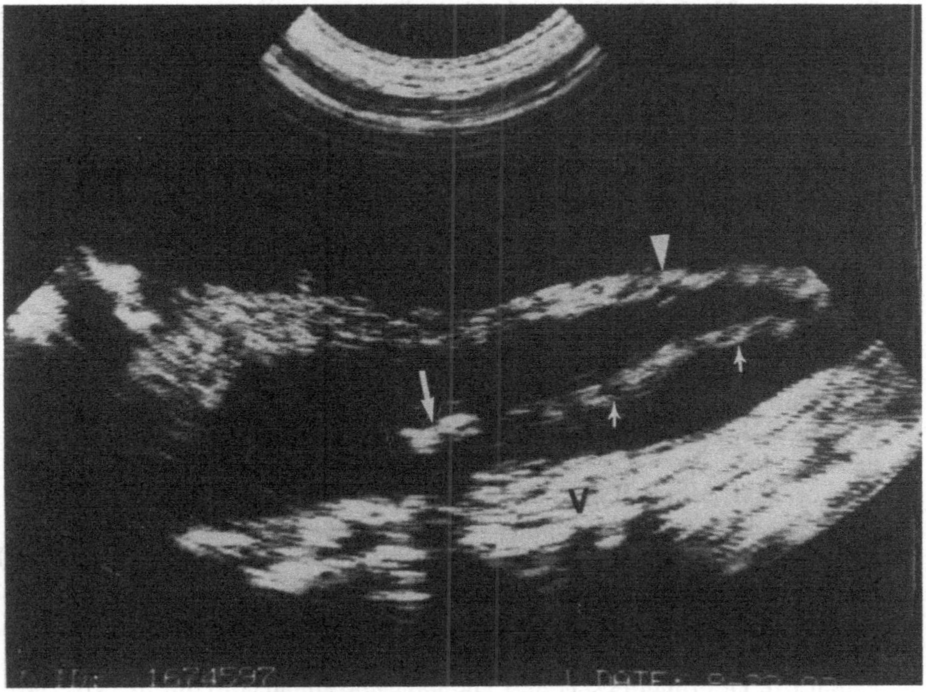


Fig. 10. Longitudinal intraoperative ultrasound scan in patient with small indriven bone fragment (arrow) within cauda equina. Nerve root (small arrows) within dural sac; posterior surface of dura (arrowhead); vertebral body (*V*)

canal, repeat ultrasound imaging would be done to check whether the spinal cord and/or cauda equina had been completely decompressed.

Indriven bone fragments or foreign bodies (such as bullet fragments) can be precisely located prior to opening the dura and may be removed with the least possible manipulation of the spinal cord or cauda equina (Fig. 10).

## VI. Summary

Intraoperative ultrasound imaging is a dynamic technique that is of value in neurotraumatology. The ultrasound scanner can be used as an instrument in the neurosurgical operating room to localize hematomas and bone fragments/foreign bodies within the central nervous system and, following removal of these, it can be used to check to see that the operation was as effective in dealing with these lesions as the neurosurgeon thought. As such it is very useful in the operative treatment of patients with injuries to the brain, spinal cord or cauda equina.

## References

1. Dohrmann GJ, Rubin JM (1981) Use of ultrasound in neurosurgical operations: a preliminary report. Surg Neurol 16: 362–366
2. Dohrmann GJ, Rubin JM (1982) Intraoperative ultrasound imaging of the spinal cord: syringomyelia, cysts and tumors. A preliminary report. Surg Neurol 18: 395–399
3. Dohrmann GJ, Rubin JM (1985) Intraoperative real-time ultrasonography: localization,characterization and instrumentation of lesions of brain and spinal cord. In: Fasano VA (ed) Advanced intraoperative technologies in neurosurgery. Springer, Wien New York, pp 3–19
4. Dohrmann GJ, Rubin JM (1985) Dynamic intraoperative imaging and instrumentation of brain and spinal cord using ultrasound. Neurol Clin 3: 425–437
5. Dohrmann GJ, Rubin JM (1985) Intraoperative diagnostic ultrasound. In: Wilkins RH, Rengachary SS (eds) Neurosurgery. McGraw-Hill, New York, pp 457–463
6. Quencer RM, Morse BM, Green BA, Eismont FJ, Brost P (1984) Intraoperative spinal sonography: adjunct to metrizamide CT in the assessment and surgical decompression of posttraumatic spinal cord cysts. AJR 142: 593–601
7. Rubin JM, Dohrmann GJ (1983) Intraoperative neurosurgical ultrasound in the localization and characterization of intracranial masses. Radiology 148: 519–524
8. Rubin JM, Dohrmann GJ (1985) The spine and spinal cord during neurosurgical operations: real-time ultrasonography. Radiology 155: 197–200
9. Rubin JM, Dohrmann GJ (1985) Efficacy of intraoperative US for evaluating intracranial masses. Radiology 157: 509–511
10. Rubin JM, Dohrmann GJ (1985) Intraoperative sonography of the spine and spinal cord. Review article. Semin Ultrasound CT MR 6: 48–67

# The Clinical Value of Multimodality Spinal Cord Evoked Potentials in the Prognosis of Spinal Cord Injury

T. TSUBOKAWA

Nihon University, School of Medicine, Tokyo (Japan)

With 10 Figures

**Contents**



## 1. Introduction

It is well known that there are various degrees of actual spinal cord damage among pateints diagnosed as having a clinically complete traumatic transectic spinal cord transection. It is important to ascertain the actual damaged area in such patients, and also in those with an incomplete spinal cord injury[7]. The recognition of the location and severity of the damaged area and its extent as related to the anatomical structure of the spinal cord is of considerable practical value to provide additional information to assist in clinical management and concerning the prognosis for the likelihood of recovery of sensory and motor disturbances, beyond what is available by careful clinical neurological examination. It also sometimes gives information to help in the selection of treatment.

For this purpose, the cortical somatosensory evoked potential (cortical SEP) has been extensively used in spinal cord injuries (Perot[12, 13], Young[25], Roward *et al.*[16]). Perot[13] reported that there was a good correlation between the alteration of the cortical SEP and the possibility of functional recovery. In some cases, the absence of the cortical SEP is indicative of a complete spinal cord lesion without any anticipated recovery of function, while its presence indicates that the injury may be incomplete with possible subsequent recovery of sensory and/or motor function (Rowed[17], Rowed *et al.*[16], Young[25]).

On the other hand, there is also evidence to suggest that the presence of the cortical SEP is not always associated with any recovery of motor function (York *et al.*[24]). This might be true, because the cortical SEP mainly reflects the function of the dorsal column in the spinal cord (Cohen *et al.*[3], Cusick *et al.*[4]), and its generator sources are quite obscure. In addition, the cortical SEP is also affected by dysfunction of the supraspinal nervous system. Therefore, the cortical SEP is not a universal indicator of the condition of the spinal cord, although many clinical reports suggest a strong positive correlation between the alteration of the initial SEP and neurological grade or quantitative prognostic information (Young[25], Rowed[17], Perot[13]). In 1976, Perot[12] insisted on recording and evaluating the descending spinal motor pathways in addition to the cortical SEP recording for electrophysiological testing of the functional integrity of long spinal cord pathways in patients with cord injury.

In order to check the various kinds of conduction or activity of the spinal cord, not only the cortical SEP, but also various kinds of evoked potential recording in the spinal cord including pyramidal motor responses (Levy *et al.*[8, 9], Tsubokawa *et al.*[21, 22]) have to be recorded in the acute stage of spinal cord injury. But it is important to select evoked potentials that have clear generator sources and records at the oligolynaptic neuronal structure.

In our clinic, we have selected segmental spinal cord evoked potentials (segmental SEP), conductive spinal cord evoked potentials (conductive SEP) and cortico-spinal descending evoked potentials (CDSEP: pyramidal potentials or corticopetal potential) or transcranially descending evoked spinal cord potentials (TDSEP: centrifugal descending potentials) as multimodality evoked spinal cord potentials.

This paper presents the methods for recording multimodality spinal cord evoked potentials. Their neurophysiological basis and clinical significance in the evaluation of the severity of spinal cord injury are also presented. As regards the clinical significance, the following matters are discussed: (1) how reliably do the multimodality spinal cord evoked potentials correlate with neurological evidence of dysfunction, and (2) how well can the multimodality spinal cord evoked potentials predict the prognosis of a cord lesion as compared with the cortical SEP and neurological examination.

## 2. Recording Methods of the Multimodality Spinal Cord Evoked Potentials in Acute Spinal Cord Injury

### *2.1. Timing of Recording of the Multimodality Evoked Potentials*

When a patient suspected of having a spinal cord injury arrives at the emergency room, the same priorities as are established for the accident scene must be initiated: both respiratory and cardiovascular stabilization and immobilization of the entire spine in a neutral spine position.

Following neurological examination, both the location of the level of injury and the severity of the damage are evaluated using the Sunnybrook's injury scales[19] (Table 1). And various kinds of fixation after radiological examination has to apply. Before carrying out emergency surgical treatment, for the prediction of functional recovery of the damaged spinal cord the stimulating and recording electrodes are set up to record the multimodality spinal cord evoked potentials. Recording and analysis of these potentials are begun, and these potentials are sporadically recorded during emergency surgery or the application of Halo-devices for early restoration of vertebral column alignment and early rigid immobilization of the spinal column. All recording systems are removed three to four days after the injury.

### *2.2. Electrode Placement*

During the X-ray examination, just after the neurological examination, 18-gauge Touhy needles are inserted into the epidural space at levels, two to five vertebrae both above and below the suspected cord injury level. A flexible insulated platinum electrode (Fig. 1) (0.9 mm in diameter: PISCES. M-8483. Medtronic Co) with a bare tip (1.5 mm in length), is inserted through the Touhy needle to about one or two vertebral spaces close to the lesion beyond the tip of the Touhy needle. After insertion of the electrodes, their locations are checked by X-ray, and the Touhy needles are removed (Fig. 2). These electrodes are used as active electrodes, to record spinal cord evoked responses and can also be used as spinal cord stimulating electrodes. An indifferent electrode is inserted into the paravertebral muscle at the same levels as the tip of active electrodes (Fig. 2).

Table 1. *The Evaluation of Severity of the Damage by Neurological Examination (Sunnybrook's Injury Scale*[16]*)*

A. Neurological Grade: The Sunnybrook Scale of the Severity of the Neurological Injury

| Grade | description |
|---|---|
| 1 | Complete motor loss. Complete sensory loss. |
| 2 | Complete motor loss. Incomplete sensory loss. |
| 3 | Incomplete motor useless. Complete sensory loss. |
| 4 | Incomplete motor useless. Incomplete sensory loss. |
| 5 | Incomplete motor useless. Normal sensory. |
| 6 | Incomplete motor useful. Complete sensory loss. |
| 7 | Incomplete motor useful. Incomplete sensory loss. |
| 8 | Incomplete motor useful. Normal sensory. |
| 9 | Normal motor. Incomplete sensory loss. |
| 10 | Normal motor. Normal sensory. |

B. Clinical Neurological Status: Method for Assessing Neurological Deficit

| Motor power* | | Sensation** | |
|---|---|---|---|
| Grade | description | Grade | description |
| 0 | No contraction | 0 | Absent (all dermatomes below injury) |
| 1 | Flicker of movement | 1 | Incomplete or patchy |
| 2 | Active movement/gravity eliminated | 2 | Normal |
| 3 | Active movement vs gravity | | |
| 4 | Active movement vs slight resistance | | |
| 5 | Active movement vs moderate resistance | | |
| 6 | Active movement vs strong resistance | | |
| 7 | Normal power | | |

* Mean for all muscle groups distal to injury.
** Light touch, pon-prick, position sense.

The other stimulating electrodes are applied to the skin overlying the tibial nerve in the popliteal fossa, and also over the median nerve using a bipolar surface electrode (Fig. 3 E). Stimulating electrodes of the cortico-spinal descending evoked potentials (CDSEP), consist of a pair of screw

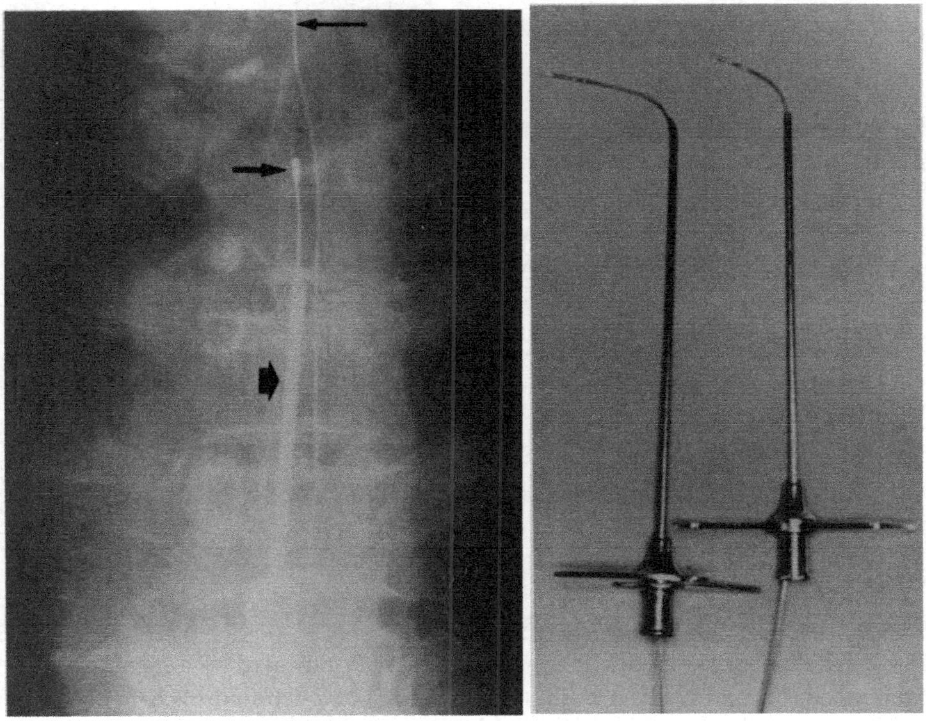

Fig. 1 The insertion of flexible insulated platinum electrode through the Touhy epidural anesthetic needle. On the right side, two sets of electrodes have been inserted through the Touhy needle and the electrode at the cranial level to the spinal cord injury has been inserted (indicated by the thin long arrow), and the other electrode (indicated by long arrow) is inserted through the Touhy needle (indicated by thick short arrow) on the left side

electrodes, which are silver-centered screws coated with ceramic (diameter 2 mm); these are twisted into the skull at a region, which is 2.0 cm posterior to bregma and 3–5 cm lateral to the midline, corresponding to the motor area, using a twist drill under local anesthesia (Fig. 3 B). Instead of using screw electrodes, a pair of needle electrodes is inserted into the scalp at a site region, 2.0 cm posterior to bregma and 3–6 cm lateral to the sagittal plane, corresponding to the motor area (Fig. 3 A), are used in some patients as stimulating electrodes for transcranial evoked descending spinal cord potentials (TDSEP).

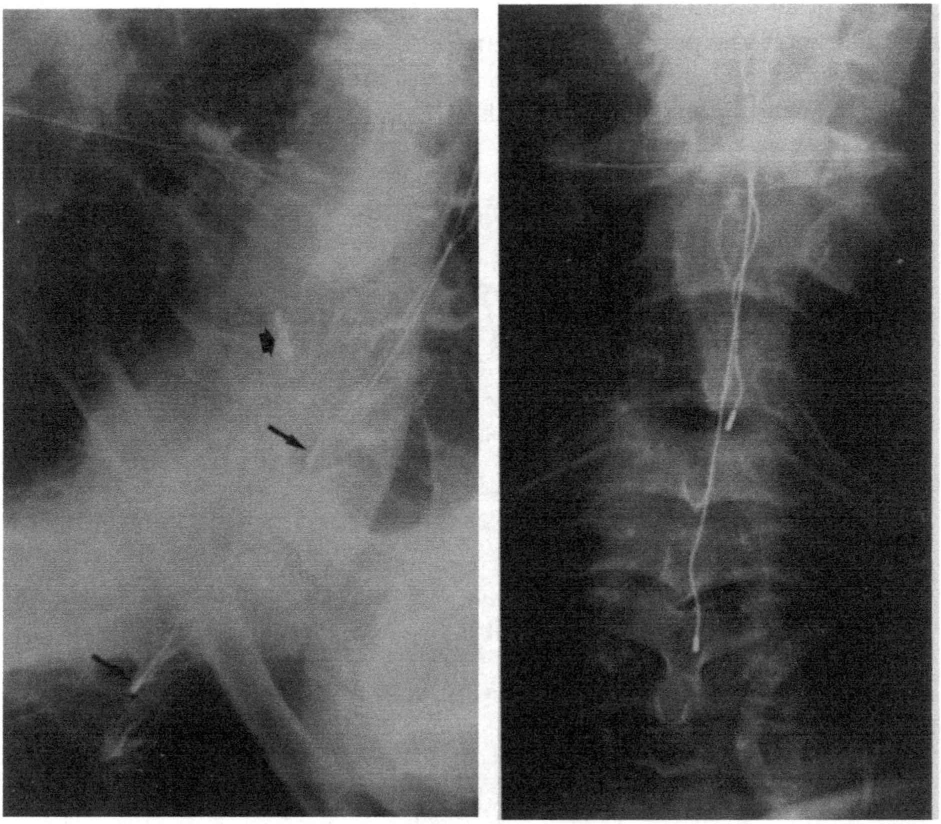

Fig. 2. The tips of electrodes at the epidural space (indicated by long arrow) have been set above and below the injured cord, are demonstrated by X-ray. And an indifferent needle electrode (indicated by large arrow) has been inserted into the paravertebral muscle at the same level of the tip of active electrode

### *2.3. Recording Methods*

The multimodality spinal evoked potentials mainly consist of four types of evoked responses: segmental SEP, conductive SEP, CDSEP and TDSEP, depending upon selection of adequate stimulation and recording electrode as in the following description (Fig. 3).

(1) recording of segmental SEP:

The segmental SEP can be recorded from the epidurally inserted electrode at the entry zone in response to stimulation of the peripheral nerve. The stimulation range of the peripheral nerve is 1.0–0.5 msec rectangular pulses and at the intensity which is a supramaximal stimulus observed on the muscle with a threshold to ensure that we obtain adequate activation of the peripheral nerve (Fig. 3).

Table 2. *The Alteration of Conductive SEP and Motor Outcome of the Cord Injured Cases*. No patient had any recovery of motor function, if both $N_1$ and $N_2$ could not recorded in the acute stage, on the other hand, not all patients had recovery of motor functions, if both $N_1$ and $N_2$ were recorded with low amplitude and simple wave

| Pretreatment | | Motor outcome |
|---|---|---|
| Conductive SEP | No. of cases | |
| Flat-potential $N_1$ and $N_2$ | 3 cases | 3/3 No recovery |
| Flat potential-traceable record $N_1$ or $N_2$ | 6 cases | 2/6 No recovery<br>3/6 need help for stand<br>1/6 able to walk |
| Low amplitude simple wave $N_1$ and $N_2$ | 6 cases | 2/6 No recovery<br>2/6 need help for stand<br>2/6 able to walk |

(2) recording of conductive SEP:

The conductive SEP (Figs. 3 C–D, D–C) can be recorded from one of the epidurally inserted electrodes that responds to stimulation of the spinal cord by using the other epidural electrode (0.3–0.5 msec, 3–10 mA rectangular pulse). When stimulation is applied to the rostral side electrode, the descending responses can be recorded by the caudal electrode, and the ascending response is recorded by the rostral epidural spinal cord electrode following caudal spinal cord stimulation.

(3) recording of pyramidal potentials (CDSEP) by direct cortical stimulation:

The motor cortex is stimulated by a pair of screw electrodes (0.3–0.5 msec duration, 10–30 mA rectangular pulse triggered by the R spike of the ECG), and the evoked potentials are recorded by both the superior (nostral) and inferior (caudal) epidural electrodes which are inserted epidurally both above and below the site of injury of the spinal cord (Fig. 3 B–C).

(4) recording of descending spinal cord evoked potential (TDSEP):

These potentials can be recorded by using epidural spinal electrodes in response to scalp stimulation. The intensity of stimulation to induce the evoked potentials is quite high as compared with direct cortical stimulation.

Stimulation is for 0.3–0.5 msec duration and with more than a 30 mA intensity rectangular pulse (Fig. 3A–C).

All evoked responses are recorded by the conventional evoked response averager (64–128 sweeps) for clinical use. The time constant of the amplifier

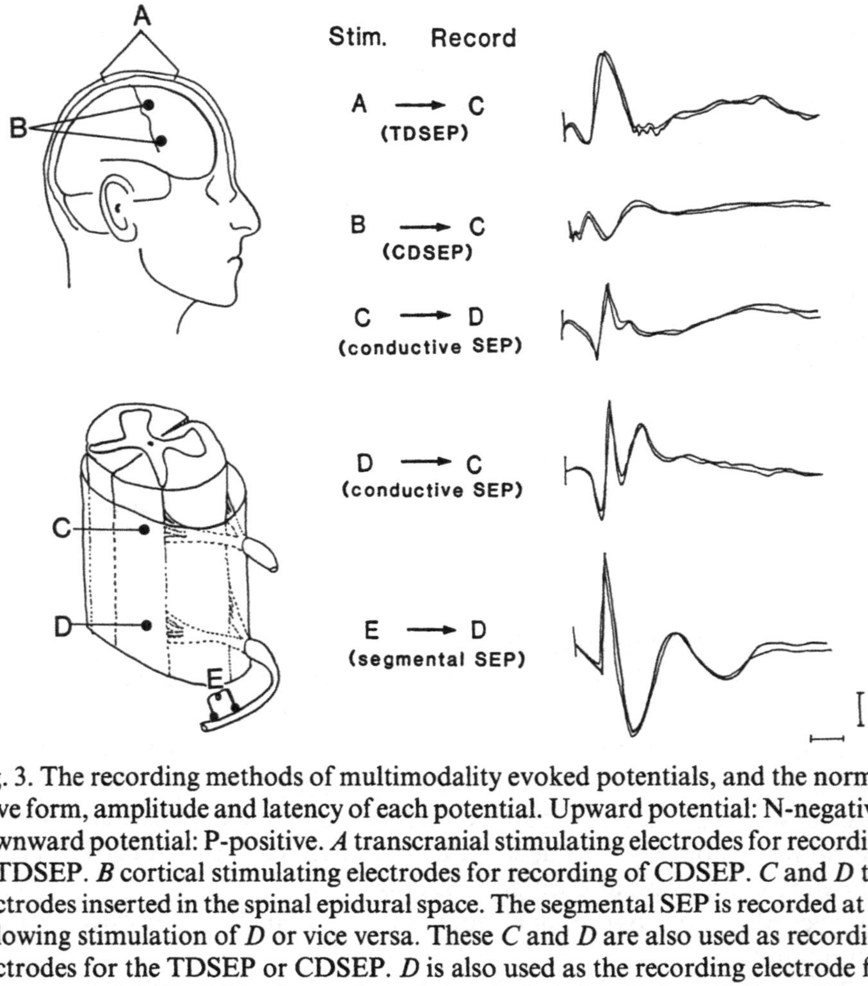


Fig. 3. The recording methods of multimodality evoked potentials, and the normal wave form, amplitude and latency of each potential. Upward potential: N-negative, downward potential: P-positive. *A* transcranial stimulating electrodes for recording of TDSEP. *B* cortical stimulating electrodes for recording of CDSEP. *C* and *D* the electrodes inserted in the spinal epidural space. The segmental SEP is recorded at *C*, following stimulation of *D* or vice versa. These *C* and *D* are also used as recording electrodes for the TDSEP or CDSEP. *D* is also used as the recording electrode for the segmental SEP. *E* Bipolar surface electrode for stimulation of the peripheral nerve (posterior tibial or median nerve). Calibration; TDSEP 1 μV, 2 m/sec. CDSEP 10 μV, 5 m/sec. Conductive SEP 50 μV, 2 m/sec. Segmental SEP 5 μV, 10 m/sec

sets 0.3 msec and the high cut at 1 kHz and the low cut at 5 Hz is used, the stimulations are triggered by the R spike of the electrocardiogram. And amplification, number of responses according to stimulus rate and intensities are standardized. Recording of each evoked potential is repeated at least three times to monitor the intrinsic variability of the evoked responses.

### 2.4. Neurophysiological Bases of each Spinal Evoked Potentials

#### 2.4.1. Segmental SEP

The wave patterns of the potentials in normal controls show a positive ($P_1$), negative ($N_1$) and positive wave ($P_2$) configuration (Fig. 3 E–D). The $P_1$ wave is a mono- or polyphasic spike potential that represents an afferent

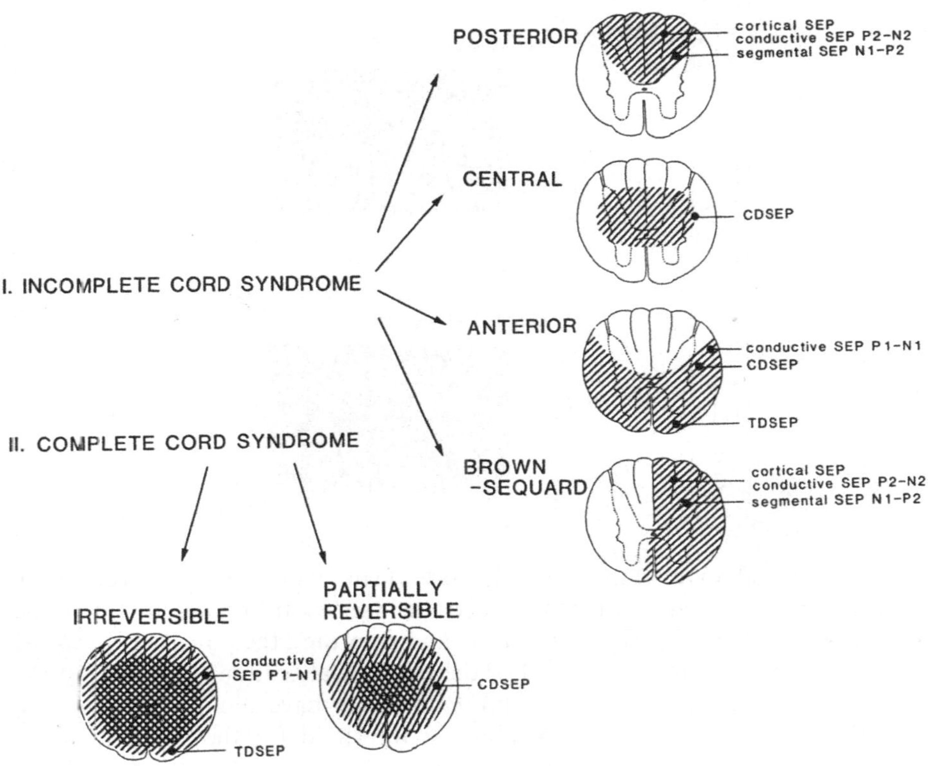


Fig. 4. The location of spinal cord injury and the affected evoked potentials

volley conducted through the dorsal root fibers. The $N_1$ component has the highest peak potential, and it is followed by the slow positive $P_2$ component (Fig. 3). Both $N_1$ and $P_2$ are generated at the dorsal horn. The alteration of these responses can indicate the disturbance of conduction, excitability of the dorsal root or dysfunction in the dorsal horn at the level of the entry zone belonging to the stimulated peripheral nerve (Fig. 4). Analysis of the segmental SEP is mainly able to identify the degree and extension of the injured area of the dorsal root and dorsal horn. In patients where the cortical SEP disappears completely after spinal cord injury, there are, at least three types of injury: The first is the lesion located in the dorsal column (posterior type of incomplete injury), the second is the lesion located in the dorsal root or dorsal horn root (a kind of central lesion or compression) and the third is a complete transecting lesion. These three types of the lesion can be differentiated by an analysis of the segmental SEP with the cortical SEP. By using other segmental SEP and CDSEP, the degree and extension of the lesion is also clearly identified (Fig. 4).

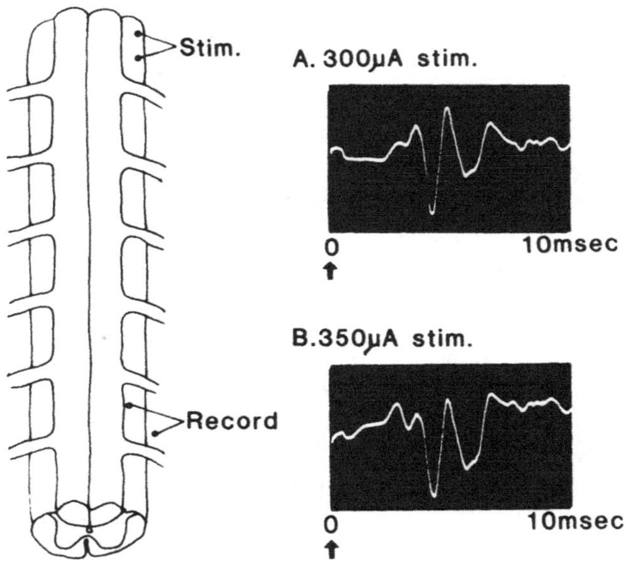


Fig. 5. The normal waves of the segmental SEP. *A* stimulate at the cranial electrode and recording the potentials from the electrode inserted at the caudal level of the injury. *B* stimulate at the caudal electrode and recording the potentials from the electrode inserted at the cranial level of the injury. Calibration; 10 m/sec, 50 μV. The potentials record by using *A* and *B* methods have almost similar wave configuration, but there is a slightly higher threshold for the stimulation for recording on *B*

### 2.4.2. Conductive SEP

The normal conductive SEP shows a positive ($P_1$), negative ($N_1$) and positive ($P_2$) and negative ($N_2$ configuration (Fig. 3). These responses show completely the same configurations of both $N_1$ and $N_2$, whether the stimulation is applied to the rostral or caudal electrode (Figs. 3 and 5, 6) in the normal cases.

The $P_1$ and $N_1$ waves are action potentials from the lateral funiculi, which has a 75 m/sec conduction velocity, and $P_2$–$N_2$ are action potentials from the dorsal columns, which has a 55 m/sec conduction velocity. The alteration of the conductive SEP indicates the disturbance of conductivity through the lateral column and dorsal column. The recording of conductive

SEP as a monitor for estimation of the function of the lateral ($N_1$-wave) and dorsal column ($N_2$-wave) has been used in spinal cord injury patients and in relation to spinal cord surgery. In our clinic, the alterations of amplitude of both $N_1$ and $N_2$ waves have been studied with relation to recovery of the motor and sensory function as shown in Fig. 5 and Table 3. Recovery of the motor function of patients who had no potentials (both $N_1$ and $N_2$), could not be expected. On other hand, motor function did not always recover, if

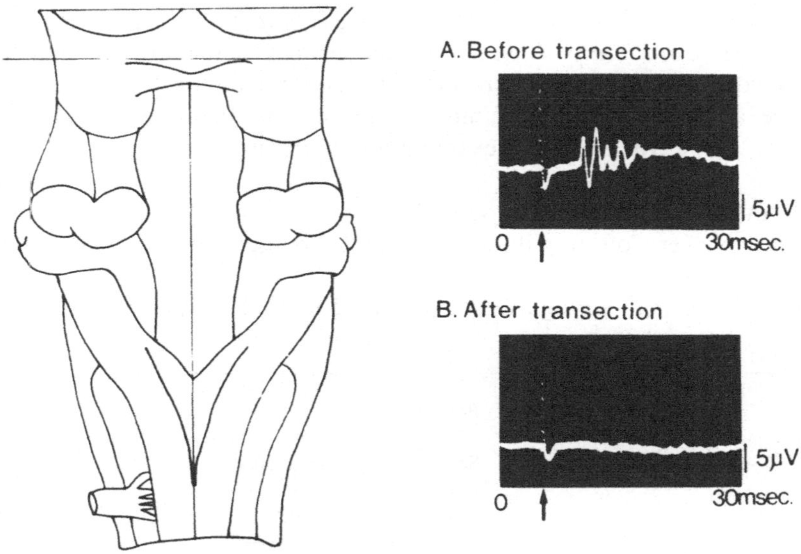


Fig. 6. The CDSEP has completely disappeared after transection at the inter-collicular level of the midbrain (cat). Calibration; 5 μV, 30 m/sec

both $N_1$ and $N_2$ waves could be recorded in the spinal cord injured cases. Therefore it might be concluded that there was not strong positive correlation between function and changes in the responses, except when both $N_1$ and $N_2$ disappear (Fig. 5 and Table 3).

The conductive SEP is able to detect the conductivity of the lateral ($N_1$) and dorsal columns ($N_2$), which might give information about the extension of a central cord lesion or a dorsal cord lesion. But it does not directly indicate the function of the pyramidal tract (Fig. 4), without recording of the CDSEP.

### 2.4.3. CDSEP (Pyramidal Potentials recorded at the Spinal Epidural Space)

The configuration of normal potentials shows simple positive-negative waves (D waves: conduction velocity 69–50 m/sec) followed by several waves (I waves) (Fig. 3). The D wave shows a consistent pattern even under deep anesthesia, but the I waves are not consistent in amplitude and latency and quickly disappear following the administration of an anesthetic drug. Therefore, only the D wave was investigated in the present study. The amplitude of the D wave becomes smaller the more caudal the recording. This potential indicates the activities of the pyramidal tract, according to our experimental and clinical studies (Tsubokawa *et al.*[21, 22], Yamamoto

Table 3. *Changes in the Multimodality Evoked Potentials in Patients with a Complete Spinal Cord Injury*. The relationship between changes in the multimodality spinal cord evoked potentials recorded at both pre and post treatment in the acute stage and the outcome of motor and sensory functions evaluated by neurological examination is presented

− No evoked potentials recorded (absent).

± Traceable very low amplitude with simple configuration of the potential by stronger stimulation.

\+ Almost normal configuration of the potentials with or without low amplitude or longer latency.

| Name | Age | Location of injury (complication) | Pretreatment | | | | | | |
|---|---|---|---|---|---|---|---|---|---|
| | | | Segmental SEP | | | Conduction SEP | | Cortically evoked SEP (D-wave) CDSEP | Transcranially evoked SEP (initial-wave) TDSEP |
| | | | $P_1$ | $N_1$ | $P_2$ | $P_1N_1$ | $P_2N_2$ | | |
| K. M. | 11 | C 5.6 | − | − | − | − | − | | − |
| M. T. | 31 | C 5.6.7 | − | − | − | − | − | | − |
| K. O. | 46 | C 3.4 (Head injury) | − | − | − | − | − | | − |
| A. O. | 22 | C 5 (Head injury) | − | − | − | − | − | − | − |
| S. K. | 66 | C 4.5.6 | − | − | − | − | − | − | − |
| M. K. | 22 | C 4.5.6. | ± | − | − | − | − | | − |
| Y. S. | 45 | C 4.5.6. | − | − | − | ± | ± | | ± |
| M. N. | 26 | C 4 | + | ± | ± | + | ± | | ± |
| K. H. | 29 | C 5 (Head injury) | ± | − | − | ± | − | ± | |
| S. Y. | 45 | C 5.6 | + | ± | − | + | ± | ± | |

*et al.*[23]). In order to demonstrate the relationship between the alteration of the D wave of CDSEP and pyramidal motor function, we studied fifteen patients who had a brain tumor located or infiltrating the capsula interna. After removal of the tumor, patients in whom the D wave disappeared, had complete hemiplegia, and those with a preserved D wave did not show any motor disturbance. But patients had a transient hemiparesis, if the amplitude of the D wave decreased by 50% and the latency increased to more than 10%. Therefore it is concluded that the disappearance of the D wave of the CDSEP indicates complete damage of the pyramidal tract. Experimentally, the CDSEP disappeared after transection at the intercollicular level (Fig. 6).

*Table 3 (continued)*

| Treatment in acute stage | Just after treatment in the acute stage | | | | | | | Neurological improvement or deterioration | | |
|---|---|---|---|---|---|---|---|---|---|---|
| | Segmental SEP | | | Conduction SEP | | Cortically evoked SEP (D-wave) CDSEP | Transcranially evoked SEP (initial-wave) TDSEP | Neurological score | Motor power (post) | Sensory (post) |
| | $P_1$ | $N_1$ | $P_2$ | $P_1N_1$ | $P_2N_2$ | | | pre post | | |
| laminectomy & cooling | – | – | – | – | – | | – | 1 → 1 | 0 | 1 |
| laminectomy, cooling, verterectomy & fusion | – | – | – | – | – | | – | 1 → 2 | 1 | 1 |
| laminectomy, cooling, verterectomy & fusion | + | – | – | – | – | – | – | 1 → 1 | 0 | 0 |
| laminectomy, cooling, verterectomy & fusion | – | – | – | – | – | – | – | 1 → 1 | 0 | 1 |
| Halo-device | + | ± | – | – | ± | – | | 1 → 2 | 0 | 1 |
| Halo-device | – | – | – | – | – | – | – | 1 → 1 | 0 | 1 |
| laminectomy, cooling, verterectomy & fusion | + | ± | ± | ± | + | | ± | 1 → 3 | 3 | 1 |
| laminectomy, cooling, verterectomy & fusion | + | + | ± | – | ± | | + | 1 → 6 | 6 | 2 |
| laminectomy, cooling, verterectomy & fusion | + | + | + | + | ± | ± | | 1 → 5 | 5 | 1 |
| laminectomy, cooling, verterectomy & fusion | + | + | ± | – | ± | + | | 1 → 7 | 5 | 1 |

2.4.4. TDSEP (Transcranial Descending Spinal Cord Evoked Potentials)

These potentials can be recorded by epidural spinal electrodes in response to scalp stimulation. The normal potential configuration of the TDSEP consists also of a D wave and I waves quite similar to CDSEP

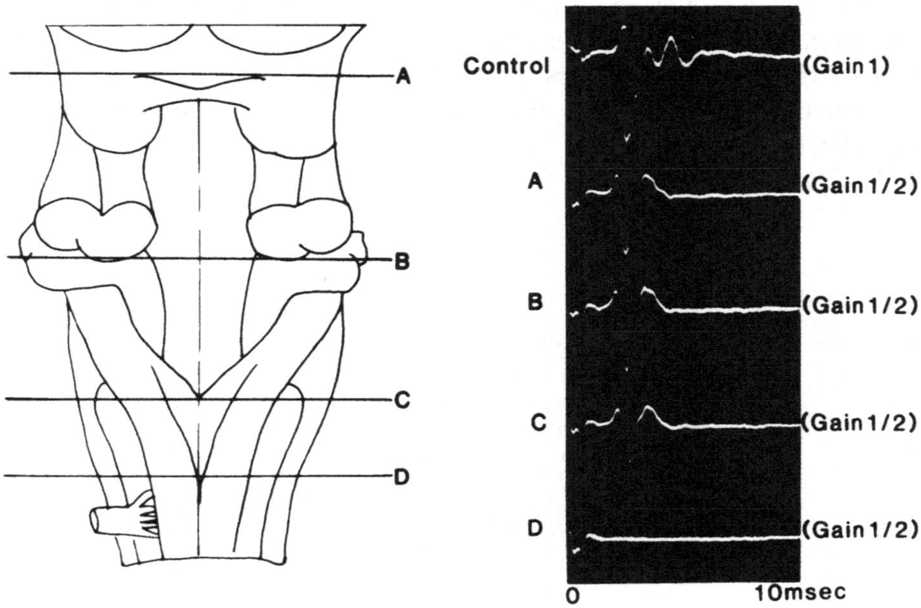


Fig. 7. The alteration of TDSEP after transection of various levels of the brainstem in animal experiments. After the transection at intercollicular level, the D wave of TDSEP is apt to increase its amplitude with decrease of I waves. The D wave or TDSEP completely disappears after transection of the medulla oblongata at the level of the obex. These facts indicate that the transcranial stimulation activates some bulbo-spinal descending tracts, like the vestibulo-spinal, reticulo-spinal and cerebello-spinal tracts. Therefore it is difficult to know if the lesion is on the left or right side of the brain in experimental animals, but it is a nice indicator in the spinal cord to know the conductivity of the ventral or ventrolateral column. Calibration; 5 μV, 10 m/sec

responses in humans. However, the animal experiment provided some inconsistant results. The conduction velocity of the initial wave of the TDSEP in cats is 90–80 m/sec, which is faster than that of the CDSEP, and the initial wave of the TDSEP is conducted, downward through the ventral and ventrolateral columns of the cord (Figs. 3 and 4). Its generating structure might be related to the vestibulospinal, reticulospinal or cerebellospinal tract according to the results of our animal experiments (Fig. 7). There is not yet conclusive data indicating that alteration of TDSEP in humans indicates the function of the pyramidal tract, we, however, tentarively consider that TDSEP in humans, in contrast to TDSEP in experimental animals, may reflect functions of pyramidal tract because of its similarty to CDSEP in the carfigulation and the latency. It is difficult to clearly record TDSEP at the cervical level because of large artifacts due to the current spread.

### 3. Interpretation of the Multimodality Evoked Potentials

In order to make a quantitative analysis of the cortical SEP, Rowed *et al.*[16] classified the alteration of the cortical SEP configuration as follows; scale 0, absent SEP: scale 1, grossly abnormal; scale 2, slightly abnormal; scale 3, normal recording. However, this scoring does not have any significant correlation with the actual spinal cord pathology, because the cortical SEP is affected by the activity of the thalamus and cortex, and does not only indicate the conductivity of the dorsal column of the spinal cord.

With an increase in clinical experience, it has become clear that the absence of the cortical SEP immediately after acute spinal cord injury correlates with severe pathological damage and a poor prognosis for subsequent clinical recovery, while the presence of a recognizable SEP has been an encouraging prognostic feature, particularly, if the $P_1$ and $N_1$ waves of the cortical SEP are either recognizable at that time or return shortly thereafter and progressively increase in amplitude.

Some investigators (Dorfman *et al.*[5, 6]) have attached more importance to latency variation, although the latencies of $P_1$ and $N_1$ of the cortical SEP are decided not only by the conductivity of the spinal cord, but are also more affected by dysfunction of the thalamic and cortical system. Others (Young[21]) have emphasized amplitude variation, although amplitude is decided by the activities of the thalamocortical system.

Analysis of spinal cord evoked potentials also involves the same problems, but these are different from the difficulties using cortical SEP, because the generating source is relatively clear and the activities are not related to many synapses and are not affected by the activity of supraspinal neural tissue. Concerning these potentials, it is difficult to set a common standard of the peak-to-peak amplitude of each potential, because the distance between the recording electrode and the spinal cord is not constant. But the latency and conduction velocity of the spinal cord evoked potentials are constant in normal subjects. We can also compare the changes of amplitude in the CDSEP, TDSEP and conductive SEP, because of the difference of amplitude of evoked potentials recorded both above and below the spinal cord injury comparisons are possible by using our CDSEP, TDSEP and conductive SEP.

Therefore, we evaluated the multimodality evoked responses as follows:

(1) absent, (2) traceable very-low amplitude with simple configuration of the potential if stimulation increases, and (3) recognized potentials at the same latency as normal subjects (Fig. 8). We also studied (1) the abnormality of the latency of each potential which changed by more than 10%, and (2) the conduction velocity in conductive SEP and CDSEP or TDSEP, and compared it with normal records. Elongation of the conduction time, decrease of amplitude of potentials (by more than 50%), simplification or polarity changes of potential and disappearance of the action potential

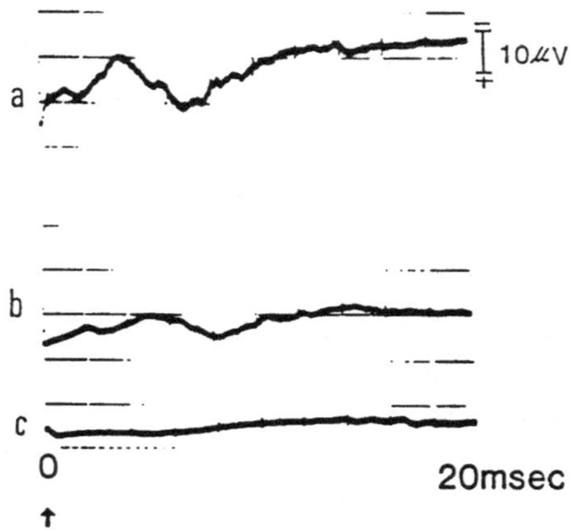


Fig. 8. The classification of the changes of each evoked potential. *a* normal wave form (amplitude and latency) of CDSEP. *b* the amplitude decreases more than 50% of normal, latency increase more than 10% and simplification of the wave configuration. *c* no response. Calibration; 10 µV, 20 m/sec. On the Tables 3 and 4, *a* is indicated by +, *b* is indicated by ± and *c* is indicated by —

clearly indicate abnormality of activity, and disappearance of the potential indicates complete conduction blocking. The cause is tissue destruction in the potential related structure of the spinal cord (Fig. 4).

If serial recording of spinal cord potentials in the acute stage of spinal cord injury is performed, the improvement or deterioration of each evoked potential can be correlated with neurological change in the three to four days following the cord injury.

**4. Clinical Assessment of Neurological Improvement or Deterioration**

We attempted to compare the results of multimodality spinal cord evoked potentials in the acute stage of spinal cord injury with the neurological state when the patient was discharged and followed up after a year (Tables 3 and 4).

In 23 patients, the multimodality spinal cord evoked potentials were recorded both before and just after treatment in the acute stage following cervical cord injury, but four died after the recording before any follow-up neurological examination could be made.

Ten were neurologically diagnosed as having a complete cord injury with complete paraplegia, although this was not certain in 3 patients, because they were unconscious from an associated head injury (Table 3).

Nine other cases were neurologically diagnosed as having incomplete cord lesion (Table 4). In the incomplete cervical cord injury group, it was difficult to identify the extent of the cord damage in four cases by neurological examination, two others were diagnosed as having central cord damage, two had a Brown-Séquard syndrome and one patient was diagnosed as having a posterior cord syndrome.

In the complete cervical cord lesion group, laminectomy and local cooling was immediately performed in eight patients, and vertebrectomy

Table 4. *Changes of the Multimodality Evoked Potentials on the Cases Suffered from Incomplete Spinal Cord Injury.* The relationship between the changes of the evoked potentials recorded at both pre and post treatment in the acute stage and the outcome of motor sensory functions by neurological examination is presented

| Name | Age | Location of injury (complication) | Pretreatment | | | | | | |
|---|---|---|---|---|---|---|---|---|---|
| | | | Segmental SEP | | | Conduction SEP | | Cortically evoked SEP (D-wave) CDSEP | Transcranially evoked SEP (initial-wave) TDSEP |
| | | | $P_1$ | $N_1$ | $P_2$ | $P_1N_1$ | $P_2N_2$ | | |
| T. O. | 23 | C 4.5 | + | + | + | − | + | − | − |
| K. N. | 19 | C 4.5 | + | + | + | − | + | − | |
| S. T. | 48 | C 5.6 (spondylosis) | + | + | − | ± | ± | | − |
| O. Y. | 18 | C 5.6 | + | + | − | ± | ± | | ± |
| K. Y. | 20 | C 5.6 | + | ± | − | + | ± | | ± |
| M. M. | 34 | C 7 | + | ± | − | − | ± | | + |
| S. N. | 30 | C 3 | + | + | − | ± | − | rt-stim. (+)<br>lt-stim. (−) | |
| M. S. | 54 | C 5.6.7 | + | − | − | ± | − | rt-stim. (−)<br>lt-stim. (+) | |
| T. T. | 55 | C 4.5 (spondylosis)<br>− | + | − | − | + | − | | + |

and fusion were undertaken in seven cases within two weeks of local cooling. Two patients were conservatively treated by application of a Halo-device.

In the incomplete cervical cord injury group, four patients were conservatively treated by application of a Halo-device, three by an anterior operation (vertebrectomy or discectomy and fusion with or without local cooling), one by laminectomy and local cooling and another by surgery to remove the laminar fracture fragment by a posterior approach (Table 4).

## 5. Results

### *Changes of Multimodality Spinal Cord Evoked Responses in Acute Cervical Cord Injury*

The multimodality spinal cord evoked potentials were completely recorded in 19 patients suffering from neurological complete and in-

*Table 4 (continued)*

| Treatment in acute stage | Just after treatment in the acute stage | | | | | | | Neurological improvement or deterioration | | |
|---|---|---|---|---|---|---|---|---|---|---|
| | Segmental SEP | | | Conduction SEP | | Cortically evoked SEP (D-wave) CDSEP | Transcranially evoked SEP (initial-wave) TDSEP | Neurological score | Motor power (post) | Sensory (post) |
| | $P_1$ | $N_1$ | $P_2$ | $P_1N_1$ | $P_2N_2$ | | | pre post | | |
| verterectomy, fusion & cooling | + | + | + | − | + | − | − | 2–5 | 3 | 2–1 |
| Halo-device | + | + | + | − | + | − | − | 4–5 | 3 | 3 |
| Discotomy & fusion | + | + | + | + | + | | − | 4–5 | 3 | 3 |
| Halo-device | + | + | ± | ± | + | | + | 4–7 | 6<br>hand skill | 2 |
| Halo-device | + | ± | − | ± | ± | | ± | 4–7 | 4 | 1 |
| verterectomy, fusion, cooling & Halo-device | + | + | − | ± | + | | + | 4–7 | 5 | 1 |
| Halo-device | + | + | − | ± | ± | rt-stim. (+)<br>lt-stim. (+) | | rt: 10–10<br>lt: 4–8 | rt-hand 7<br>lt-hand 4 | 1 |
| laminectomy, cooling & anterior fusion | + | + | + | ± | + | rt-stim. (−)<br>lt-stim. (+) | | rt: 4–4<br>lt: 6–10 | rt-hand 5<br>lt-hand 6 | 1–2 |
| removal of fracture fragment | + | − | − | + | − | | + | 6–9 | 7 | 1 |

complete cerivcal cord injury, both before and just after treatment in the acute stage (Tables 3 and 4).

Among 10 neurologically complete cord injury cases, no evoked potentials could be recognized in five (cases 1–5); in the other five (cases 6–

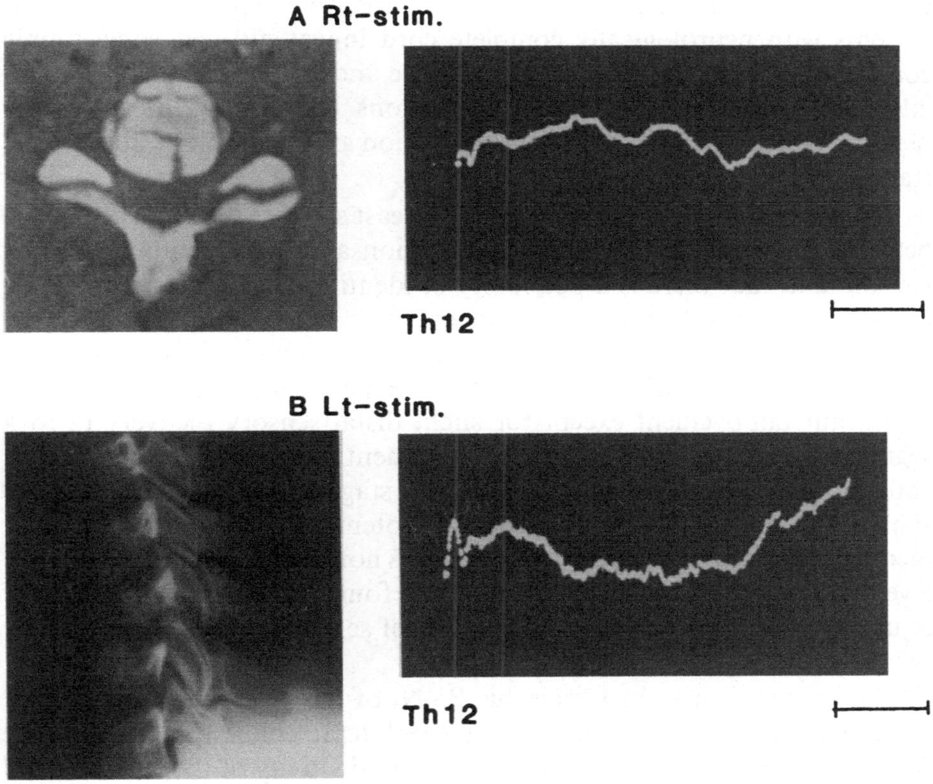


Fig. 9. TDSEP recorded in a patient with a complete spinal cord injury (case 5). No response recorded following right transcranial stimulation (*A*) and left transcranial stimulation (*B*) at $Th_{12}$ level in the epidural space. Calibration; 10 μV, 5 m/sec. CT scanning and spinal X-ray of this case are shown at left side

10), some multimodality spinal cord evoked potentials were recorded with a simple configuration of the wave form, or traceable very low amplitude with longer latency. Case 6 had only the low amplitude $P_1$ wave of the segmental SEP, but no other responses could be recorded (Fig. 9). Case 7 had also traceable responses of the $P_2$–$N_2$ potentials of the conductive SEP and TDSEP with very low amplitude and 28% increased latency, but no other responses. The $P_1$–$N_1$ waves of the segmental SEP, the $P_1$–$N_1$ of the conductive SEP and the CDSEP or TDSEP were traceably recorded with very low amplitude and 20% increased latency in cases 8, 9, and 10 (Table 2).

In patients with neurologically complete cervical cord injury, there were two patterns of multimodality spinal cord evoked potentials: the first group (cases 1–6 was that in which all spinal cord evoked responses disappeared or only the $P_1$ response of the segmental SEP was left (Fig. 4); the second group (cases 7–10) was that where components of the segmental SEP, the $P_1$–$N_1$ of the conductive SEP and CDSEP or TDSEP were reproducible. Several patients with neurologically complete cord injury still had some simple configurating potential with low amplitude and/or longer latency potentials. These findings raise serious questions concerning the difference between a neurologically complete cord lesion and a pathological complete transection of the spinal cord.

According to these results, we could at least say that there is a difference between neurologically complete cord lesion and pathoanatomical transection, and that there is a possibility of identifying some patients with a potential for neurological improvement.

Patients who did not have any spinal cord evoked potentials (cases 1–5) and the one patient with only the $P_1$ of the segmental SEP did not obtain any significant impovement except for slight distal sensory recovery (2 to 4 segments). That was, in spite of active treatment, such as laminectomy, local cooling, and/or realignment, in the early stage of the five patients who showed no activity on spinal cord evoked potentials, neurological improvement at discharge or one-year follow-up was not recognized, except that the level of sensory loss moved down to two to four segments from the level of injury. Case 6, who had only traceable $P_1$ of segmental SEP, did not show any improvement of neurological signs.

But in case 7, who had traceable $P_1$–$N_1$ of the conductive SEP, which indicated remaining conductivity of the lateral column, and traceable TDSEP, which also indicated survival of conductivity of the ventrolateral column, motor function pertially recovered (active movement against gravity) and the sensory loss level extended down six segments. This patient was different from cases 1–6 in that he had TDSEP, in spite of its amplitude being very low with a long latency.

In cases 8, 9, and 10 in the second group, traceable small amplitude and longer latency potentials, which related to the lateral column like the $P_1$–$N_1$ of the conductive SEP and CDSEP or TDSEP potentials, were recorded at pretreatment. And, after intensive treatment of these patients in the acute stage, these traceable low amplitude evoked potentials increased in amplitude, became more complex in the wave shape configuration and close to normal latency, but none of the potentials of the segmental or conductive SEP related to the posterior column or posterior horn could be recorded even after intensive treatment in the acute stage. The neurological improvement was remarkable in all three cases. Frankel's score was D at the one-year follow-up. In two of the three, active movement of both the hands was possible against moderate resistance, while the other patient was able to walk with a supporting device.

According to these findings of the multimodality spinal evoked potentials, it might be concluded that neurological improvement can be assured, whenever functions of the ventrolateral column or dorsal horn were shown to survive even slightly, by studies of the multimodality evoked potentials and those potentials increased in amplitude or became more complicated in the wave configuration following intensive treatment in the acute stage. But such neurological improvement did not always relate to the type of intensive surgical treatment in the acute stage.

Regarding the other nine cases of neurological incomplete cord injury, the multimodality spinal cord evoked potentials were recorded both before treatment and just after treatment in the acute stage. Cases 1, 2, 3, and 4 were neurologically diagnosed as having an incomplete cord injury, but the location or extent of the lesion in the cord could not be identified by neurological examination. Cases 5 and 6 were diagnosed as having central cord injury, cases 7 and 8 a Brown-Séquard type injury, and case 9 a posterior cord injury caused by fracture of the lamina.

According to the analysis of the multimodality evoked potentials in cases 1, 2, 3, and 4, the segmental SEP of cases 1 and 2 could be recorded as normal configuration potentials with a low amplitude and slight increase of the latency; the early component the $P_2$–$N_2$ of the conductive SEP was also recorded with a low amplitude, but no potentials of the $P_1$–$N_1$ of the conductive SEP and CDSEP or TDSEP could be recorded before treatment was begun. We were able to ascertain, by using the multimodality spinal evoked potentials, that these patients were suffering from anterior cord lesions. These alterations of the multimodality evoked potentials did not change following intensive treatment, i.e., vertebrectomy and fusion with local cooling in case 1, and realignment and fixation by using a Halo-device in case 2. Just after these treatments, the configuration of the multimodality spinal cord evoked potentials did not show any improvement nor any deterioration. However, neurological improvement was remarkable insofar as sensation was concerned, while motor power showed only active movement against gravity.

In the other two cases (case 3 and 4), the $P_1$–$N_1$ of the segmental SEP could be recorded with absence of the $P_2$ wave, potentials of conductive SEP showed a very low or absent amplitude and the CDSEP or TDSEP was not recorded or traceable. These alterations of the spinal cord evoked potential indicated injury of the central parts of the spinal cord (Fig. 4).

After intensive treatment in the acute stage, the amplitude of every potential increased and showed a more complex wave configuration of the segmental and conductive SEP. The TDSEP increased in amplitude in case 4, who had good recovery of motor function, but was not recorded in case 3.

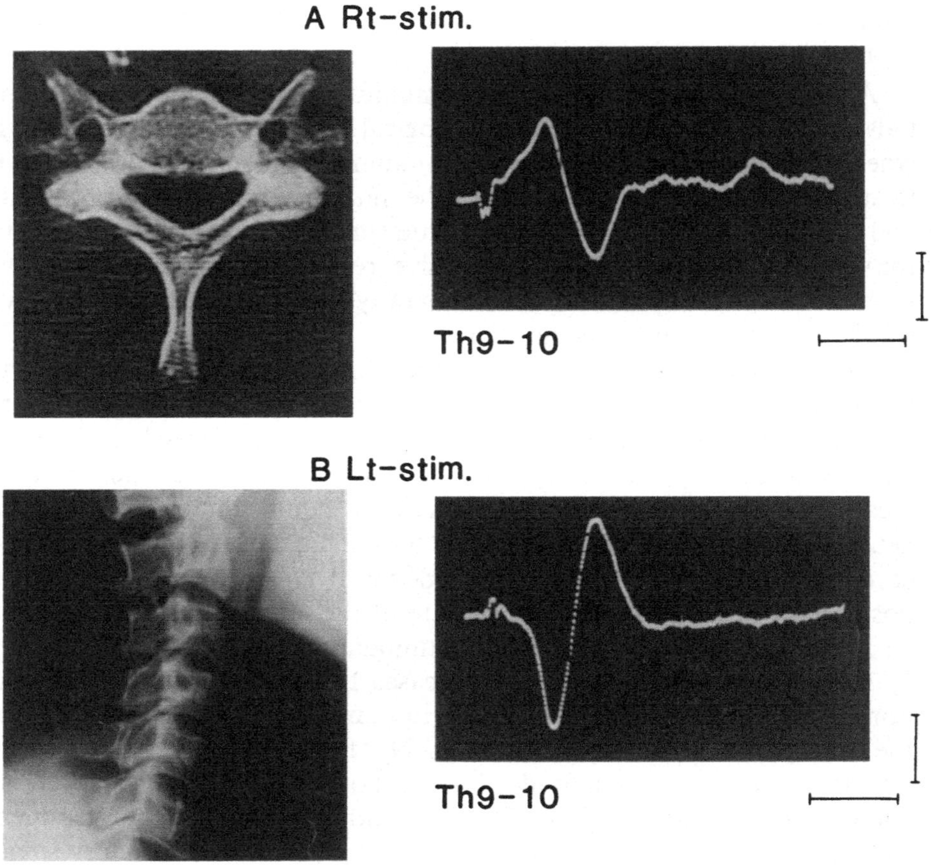


Fig. 10. The TDSEP recorded in a patient with an incomplete spinal cord injury (case 6, central cord syndrome). There is the initial potential of TDSEP recorded from the spinal epidural space at $Th_{9-10}$ level. Although the phase reversal of the D wave is observed on the left (*B*) and right side stimulation (*A*), the latency of the D wave does not differ between these two recordings. A remarkable recovery of motor function occurred in this patient. Calibration; 10 μV, 5 m/sec

In the central cord syndrome group (case 5 and 6), the $P_1$ potential of the segmental SEP was recorded, but the $N_1$–$P_1$ could not be recorded; the $P_1$–$N_1$ of the conductive SEP was recorded in case 5, in spite of the fact that traceable $P_2$–$N_2$ could be recorded in these patients. The TDSEP or CDSEP was recorded in case 6 (Fig. 10), but only a very small traceable potential with a longer latency in case 5. These patients showed findings very similar to cases 3 and 4. Therefore, they might be diagnosed as having a central cord syndrome (Fig. 4), according to the analysis of the multimodality evoked potentials.

Just after treatment in the acute stage, the amplitude became higher and the potential configuration became more complex in the segmental and conductive SEP in all cases, but there was only a slight increase in the TDSEP.

As for the Brown-Séquard type injury group (cases 7 and 8), the alterations of the segmental SEP and conductive SEP were not constant, but the $P_2$ wave of the segmental SEP and both waves of the conductive SEP could not be recorded except for traceable potentials with long latencies. The D wave of the CDSEP disappeared by stimulation of contralateral side of the hemiplegia. After treatment with a Halo-device in case 7, stimulation of the contralateral side of the hemiplegia could induce the CDSEP potential, which was low in amplitude, and this patient showed remarkable improvement of neurological signs (Table 4).

As for the patient with a posterior cord injury (case 9) the $P_2$ of the segmental SEP and the $P_2$–$N_2$ of the conductive SEP could not be recorded, but the TDSEP was recorded with a low amplitude and simple configuration. The segmental SEP and conductive SEP did not change after intensive surgical treatment involving removal of the bone fragment from the epidural space, but neurological improvement was remarkable with almost normal motor function and only slight sensory disturbance at the $C_{4-5}$ level.

According to these findings of the multimodality spinal evoked potentials, it might be concluded that, in the incomplete cord lesion group, analysis of alteration of each evoked response can demonstrate the extent or location of the pathological lesion in the spinal cord and provide information of the probability of neurological improvement at the pretreatment stage (Fig. 4).

## 6. Discussion

The multimodality spinal cord evoked response, by which the function of the posterior root and dorsal horn (analysis on the segmental SEP), the conduction of both the posterior and lateral column of the cord (analysis on conductive SEP), and centripetal conduction, including the pyramidal tract (analysis on CDSEP or TDSEP) can be checked, is useful to ascertain not only the severity, but also the location and extent of the injured area in the spinal cord by recording in acute stage of spinal cord injury. Analysis of the multimodality evoked potentials in the acute stage also enables us to know the pathological state of the cord injury, as is shown in our experimental study (Tsubokawa *et al.*[22]). The results clearly demonstrate the alteration of multimodality evoked responses between pre and post treatment in the acute stage and also indicate the possibility of neurological improvement by treatment at the acute stage.

The clinical significance of the multimodality spinal cord evoked potentials is completely different from that of cortical SER, which has been widely advocated for evaluating spinal cord injury (Dorfman *et al.*[5, 6], Perot[13], Young[25], Rowed *et al.*[16], Sedgwick *et al.*[18]). Young's study[25] suggested the following; (1) SEP is a reliable means of assessing neurological function in patients with spinal cord injury, (2) in a small percentage of patients, it may be a more sensitive method than neurological examination to detect residual sensory pathways, and acute injury is primarily manifested by changes in the amplitude of potential. There are quite strong positive findings which demonstrate the usefullness of cortical SEP recording in acute spinal cord injury. But there is no clear answer concerning the clinical evaluation of recording of cortical SEP in spinal cord injury, because its changes only indicate disturbance of the proprioceptive sensory pathway including the dorsal column. Therefore there are some aspects regarding the clinical significance of cortical SEP in patients with a spinal cord injury that are quite contraversial. The studies also suggest that the cortical SEP may have a value in patients with altered levels of consciousness, but this is also negative evidence, because the cortical SEP is markedly affected by an associated severe head injury.

Although the recording of cortical SEP is simple, not time consuming, and so a non-invasive technique, the alteration of the responses of cortical SEP does not pathophysiologically indicate the severity or location of the damaged area and it may be influenced by many other factors, such as an alteration of blood pressure, anesthesia or certain other drugs, and by an associated cerebral injury. In addition, Bennett[1] reported a valuable comparison of the cortical SEP and motor evoked potential derived from direct stimulation of the motor cortex in the cat, which indicated that a loss of descending activity was not always accompanied by a loss of ascending activity during spinal cord compression and that lesser degrees of spinal cord ischemia could produce dysfunction in the descending system. This indicates that when recording the activity of the descending system it is important to appreciate the functional disturbance induced by cord injury associated ischemic change, which is always observed in biological studies of spinal cord injury.

To obtain such information, the recording of multimodality evoked spinal cord responses, which are selected from the response related with certain tracts for both sensory and motor function, is necessary to provide an adequate clinical evaluation for spinal cord injury patients. According to our experimental study on spinal cord injury, the analysis of changes on segmental SEP, conductive SEP and pyramidal response (CDSEP) was clearly able to indicate the extension and severity of the damaged area in the spinal cord, with good correlation with the pathological findings (Tsubokawa *et al.*[22]).

For the prediction about the possibility of recovery of neurological deficit, it is important to know not only the alteration of both amplitude and latency of the each of the potentials at an early stage of spinal cord injury, but also facts about increase in amplitude or decreased latency after treatment in the acute stage, or comparing the potentials recorded above and below the lesion, because the disappearance or absence of the potentials during the treatment at the early stage, clearly demonstrates an irreversible lesion, as is shown in our results. There are still no criteria indicating how much decrease in amplitude and how much increase in latency indicate an irreversible spinal cord damage.

Concerning the safety of recording of multimodality spinal evoked potentials, there are some contraversial views [10]. When recording spinal cord evoked potentials, the electrode require to be inserted into the epidural space of the spinal cord and the brain, and electrical stimulation is applied to the spinal cord or the motor cortex through the dura in patients with an acute spinal cord injury. These techniques have been criticized as being too invasive and risky (Lueder *et al.* [10]). But the insertion of stimulating electrodes into the epidural space can be performed easily without flexion of the patient's body, or even after the application of a Halo-device by doctors who are treating spinal cord injury patients, if a flexible platinum electrode is inserted by the guide technique using a Touhy needle. Regarding direct electrical stimulation of the spinal cord or of the motor cortex, several reports have been published about the safety (Mortimer *et al.* [11], Pudenz *et al.* [15]). The effects of the electric current on neural tissue were studied by Mortimor *et al.* in an experiment that involved the application of electric current directly to the brain surface. The critical value determined in that study was 0.05 w/in$^2$, which should be modified if the current is delivered from out side the dura mater and Pudenz *et al.* also gave safety guidelines [15]. Our parameter (stimuli with a maximum strength of 15 mA, 0.3 msec is delivered) is well below these guidelines and stimulation is used intermittently with relatively long rest periods between runs, except for trans-cranial stimulation for recording TDSEP. Therefore the recording method of spinal cord evoked responses does not cause any damage to neural tissue although it is slightly invasive.

Concerning the safety of the recording of both CDSEP and TDSEP, no adverse reactions have also occurred using this technique. There was a slight increase in systemic blood pressure (less than 10 mm Hg) in only 4 patients, and no respiratory changes occurred in any patient in the series. Although a possible adverse effect of this technique may appear to be the triggering of a seizure in seizure prone patient, there has been no adverse effect on spinal cord injury patients during or subsequent to the recordings. Neither did any EEG change occur in EEG recorded cases (6 such patients).

With reference to transcranial stimulation for the recording of TDSEP, more than 30 mA electric current is often used and there are still doubts whether the potential of TDSEP indicates the function of the pyramidal tract or not, because (1) stronger stimulating electrical currents are necessary to induce the TDSEP potential, (2) spreading of the electrical current, (3) at least in the cat this centrifugal potential is not an action potential for the pyramidal tract, but the TDSEP potential is generated at the ventral and ventrolateral column of the spinal cord (Tsubokawa *et al.*[22]). Levy *et al.*[8,9] showed that transcranial stimulation as well as direct motor cortex stimulation in the experimental animal can produce a descending evoked potential that may be recorded from the spinal cord and both indicate the activity of the pyramidal tract. But these descending action potentials (CDSEP and TDSEP) have different conduction times and different characteristic changes after making the lesion of the pyramidal tract (Tsubokawa *et al.*[22]). Therefore, the potential induced by direct cortical stimulation is the action potential in the pyramidal tract, but the potential induced by transcranial stimulation in the cat is the action potential related to the conductivity of the ventral and ventrolateral columns of the spinal cord. Conclusion regarding to whether TDSEP and CDSEP in humans are identical or not awaits further investigation.

Our results show that the multimodality spinal cord evoked potentials were of value to check both the sensory system and the motor system, and more analytically to ascertain the severity of pathological damage (location extension and severity), and also the effects of treatment at the early stage without any complication or any hazard to treatment in the acute stage of spinal cord injury, even during surgery or during realignment by a Halo-device. Also to predict improvement or deterioration when patients are admitted to hospital. By using multimodality evoked potentials, patients with neurologically complete cord lesion can be differentiated; thus one group can be shown to have complete transection without any neurological improvement to be expected from future treatment; and the other group an incomplete cord injury. Neurological improvement can be anticipated in some patients when traceable potentials by the multimodality spinal cord evoked potentials increase in amplitude or change to more complex wave form following certain type of some treatment. In addition, the clinical value of the multimodality spinal cord evoked potential is that the location and extent of an incomplete cord lesion can also be more clearly estimated as is shown by our clinical results.

## 7. Conclusions

The multimodality evoked spinal cord potentials, which indicate the function of the dorsal root potential, action potential at the dorsal horn (segmental SEP), conductivity at the lateral and dorsal column of the cord (conductive SEP), centripetal action potential at the ventral and ventrolateral column of the cord (TDSEP) and action potential at the pyramidal tract (CDSEP) have a clinical significance: (1) to ascertain the location and extent of spinal cord damage more precisely than does clinical neurological examination (2) to evaluate the results of intensive treatment in the acute stage, because both the damaged area and severity of the lesion will be identified; and (3) to predict the prognosis regarding neurological improvement, according to an analysis of the multimodality evoked potentials recorded before and after treatment in the acute stage. Furthermore, the methods of recording the potentials are slightly invasive but cause no harm or hazard regarding the acute spinal cord injury, and there are no complications.

It is therefore concluded that an analysis of the multimodality evoked spinal cord potentials is useful in conjunction with the clinical evaluation concerning the extent of the injury, and to predict the clinical outcome, and it differs from other any kind of single sensory evoked potential or evoked motor potential method.

## References


1. Bannett MA (1983) Effects of compression and ischemia on spinal cord evoked potentials. Exp Neurol 80: 508–514
2. Chabot R, York DH, Watts C *et al.* (1985) Somatosensory evoked potentials evaluated in normal subjects and spinal cord injured patients. J Neurosurg 63: 544–551
3. Cohen AR, Young W, Ransohoff J (1981) Intraspinal localization of the somatosensory evoked potential. Neurosurgery 9: 157–162
4. Cusick JF, Myklebust JB, Larson SJ *et al.* (1979) Spinal cord evaluation by cortical evoked responses. Arch Neurol 36: 140–143
5. Dorfman LJ (1977) Indirect estimation of spinal cord conduction velocity in man. Electroencephalogr Clin Neurophysiol 42: 26–34
6. Dorfman LJ, Perkash I, Bosley TM *et al.* (1980) Use of cerebral evoked potentials to evaluate spinal somatosensory function in patients with traumatic and surgical myelopathies. J Neurosurg 52: 654–660
7. Frankel HC, Hancock DO, Hyslop G *et al.* (1969) The value of postural reduction in the initial management of closed injuries of the spine with paraplegia and tetraplegia. Paraplegia 7: 179–192
8. Levy WG, York DH (1983) Evoked potentials from the motor tracts in humans. Neurosurgery 12: 422–429
9. Levy WJ, York DH, McCaffrey M *et al.* (1984) Motor evoked potentials from transcranial stimulation of the motor cortex in humans. Neurosurgery 15: 287–302
10. Lueders H, Gurd A, Hahn J *et al.* (1982) A new technique for intraoperative monitoring of spinal cord function. Multichannel recording of spinal cord and subcortical evoked potentials. Spine 7: 110
11. Mortimer JJ, Shealy CN, Wheeler C (1970) Experimental nondestructive electrical stimulation of the brain and spinal cord. J Neurosurg 32: 553–559

12. Perot PL (1976) Somatosensory evoked potentials in evaluation of patients with spinal cord injury. In: Morley TP (ed) Current controverses in neurosurgery. Saunders, Philadelphia, pp 160–167
13. Perot PL Jr (1973) The clinical use of somatosensory evoked potentials in spinal cord injury. Clin Neurosurg 20: 367–381
14. Perot PL Jr, Vera CL (1982) Scalp-recorded somatosensory evoked potentials to stimulation of nerves in the lower extremities and evaluation of patients with spinal cord trauma. Ann NY Acad Sci 388: 359–368
15. Pudenz RH, Bullara LA, Jacques S *et al.* (1975) Electrical stimulation of the brain III: The neural damage model. Surg Neurol 4: 389–400
16. Rowed DW, McLean JAG, Tator CH (1978) Somatosensory evoked potentials in acute spinal cord injury; prognostic value. Surg Neurol 9: 203–210
17. Rowed DW (1982) Value of somatosensory evoked potentials for prognosis in partial cord injury. In: Tator CH (ed) Early management of acute spinal cord injury. Raven Press, New York, pp 167–180
18. Sedgwick EM, El-Negamy E, Frankel H (1980): Spinal cord potentials in traumatic paraplegia and quadriplegia. J Neurol Neurosurg Psychiatry 43: 823–830
19. Tator CH, Rowed DW, Schwartz ML (1982) Sunnybrook cord injury scales for assessing neurological injury and neurological recovery. In: Tator CH (ed) Early management of acute spinal cord injury. Raven Press, New York, pp 7–24
20. Tsubokawa T, Romsay RE (1982) Evoked responses: Use in a neurological intensive care unit. In: Green BA, Marshall LF, Gallagher TJ (ed) Intensive care for neurological trauma and disease. Academic Press, New York, pp 201–215
21. Tsubokawa T, Yamamoto T, Hirayama T *et al.* (1986) Clinical application of the cortico-spinal evoked potentials as a monitor of pyramidal function. Nihon Univ J Med 28: 1–6
22. Tsubokawa T, Katayama Y, Hirayama T *et al.* (1986) Assessment of spinal cord injury with multimodality evoked spinal cord potentials. Part 1. Localization of lesions in experimental spinal cord injury. Neuro-Orthopedics 1: 130–141
23. Yamamoto T, Tsubokawa T, Hirayama T *et al.* (1985) Noninvasive monitoring of corticospinal evoked responses from the spinal epidural space in the cat. Nihon Univ J Med 27: 17–21
24. York DH, Watts C, Raffensberger M *et al.* (1983) Utilization of somatosensory evoked cortical potentials in spinal cord injury: prognostic limitations. Spine 8: 832–839
25. Young W (1982) Correlation of somatosensory evoked potentials and neurological findings in spinal cord injury. In Tator CH (ed) Early management of acute spinal cord injury. Raven Press, New York, pp 153–165

# Treatment of Thoracic and Lumbar Spine and Spinal Cord Injuries

Y. Reynier

Clinique Neuro-chirurgicale (Professeur Robert P. Vigouroux), C.H.U. Timone, Marseille (France)

With 10 Figures

## Contents

## 1. General Data

Following the pioneering work of Sir Ludwig Guttmann great efforts and researches have been made concerning thoraco-lumbar spine and spinal cord injuries.

However, great controversy still surrounds the management of both the neurological and the bony injuries. Guttmann (1949, 1954, 1973), his pupils, and others such Bedbrook (1969), Burke *et al.* 1976), Frankel *et al.* (1969), claim that open spinal surgery has no role to play.

They focussed their attention on the important role of reduction and stabilization of the spine, and less so on the persistent presence of bone and discal fragments retropulsed into the spinal canal.

The aim of nonsurgical treatment is to restore normal anatomical alignment by "postural reduction", and permits stabilization by spontaneous interbody fusion, which occurs during a period of prolonged bedrest, 8 to 12 weeks (Hardy 1965).

A major shortcoming of this method is that any injudicious handling during the early postinjury period may cause displacement of an unstable fracture and reinjure nerve roots that still retain a high potential for recovery.

Highly motivated, vigilant, and expert nursing in a specialized spinal care unit is essential to diminish the incidence of complications.

Furthermore, hospitalization is prolonged, and intensive rehabilitation efforts must be delayed until the patient can be safely allowed out of bed.

Holdsworth (1953, 1963) shared Guttmann's opinion regarding the prime necessity for spinal stability. Regarding unstable fractures, he ensured early spinal stability by surgical stabilization and realignment of the fracture by means of internal fixation with plates bolted to the spinous processes.

This surgical attitude has been stressed by many authors, who have presented convincing evidence that secure and adequate stabilization of unstable thoracic and lumbar spine fractures promotes speedier rehabilitation, easier nursing care, and decreased complications (Böhler 1956, 1970, Dickson *et al.* 1973, Flesch *et al.* 1977, Harrington 1967, 1973, Katznelson 1969, Kaufer *et al.* 1966, Kelly *et al.* 1968, Roberts *et al.* 1970).

Guttmann and Holdsworth did not appear to fully appreciate the direct observation of the intraspinal neural structures, because the assumption was made that spinal realignment accomplishes adequate neural decompression. Sometimes, spinal stability does not occur, and progressive kyphosis may cause delayed injury to the spinal cord or cauda equina roots (Kaufer *et al.* 1966).

Early decompressive laminectomy alone, with the aim to relieve bony or discal compression has been fully discussed (Burke *et al.* 1975, Morgan *et al.* 1971). Laminectomy as an isolated procedure adds to the instability (Dickson *et al.* 1973) and is useless to decompress neural tissue when the compression lies ventrally (Bradford *et al.* 1976, Doppman *et al.* 1976).

In recent years, neurological improvement following anterior spinal decompression was described (Chengqi 1979, Gage *et al.* 1969, Larson *et al.* 1976, O'Laoire 1982, Paul *et al.* 1975).

Evidence of improved neurological function by decompressive surgical procedures and fracture reduction and stabilization, either immediate or delayed, has not been conclusive (Bradford *et al.* 1977, Flesch *et al.* 1977, Lewis and Mac Kibben 1974, Osebold *et al.* 1981). Ideed, it has been felt by most authors that the maximum neurological damage occurs at the time of injury, and the most important determinant of neural recovery is the extent of damage to the neural tissues at that time (Bedbrook 1969, Guttmann 1969).

It has also been shown that incomplete cord injury has a tendency to improve without treatment (Bohlman 1974, Frankel *et al.* 1969).

What is the most effective approach in treating thoracolumbar spine fractures? Is it conservative treatment, laminectomy alone, fusion alone (Kaufer *et al.* 1966, Lewis *et al.* 1974), or decompression of neural elements associated with stabilization of the spine? (Dickson *et al.* 1978, Schmidek *et al.* 1980, Whitesides *et al.* 1976).

Certain factors influence the concepts of treatment (Seljeskog 1982). Understandably, the peculiar neurological aspect of thoracolumbar injuries, where many patients have a combination of conus injury and injury to the roots of the cauda equina, offer a potential for recovery. Another factor influencing therapy is the development of polytomography, and more recently the use of high resolution CT scanning. CT scanning and tomography can aid immeasurably in the initial assessment of the injury, including its mechanism of production, spinal stability, and more important the dimensions of the spinal canal. This initial complete radiographic evaluation will enable a decision to be made regarding an appropriate plan of therapy.

Finally, we must consider the evolution and the development of various orthopedic techniques.

The primary goal of all treatment regimes ought to be to ultimately restore the patient to maximum functional status. Kobrine *et al.* (1978) state that for thoraco-lumbar spinal injuries with a neurological deficit, treatment is best accomplished by combining two goals: decompression of the neural elements to allow maximum neurological recovery to occur, and stabilization of the spine, which will permit early mobilization and rehabilitation. Some neurosurgeons recommend conservative treatment, claiming that surgery does not improve the final result and delays rehabilitation. On the contrary others think that to operate on spinal injuries does not only permit a better spinal static and dynamic condition, which may not be the most important feature when the neurological deficit persists but may also permit more rapid mobilization of the patient. It is essential not to restrict consideration of surgery to a systematic laminectomy, but to consider modern surgical techniques, and the possible indications are assisted by information given by modern techniques of investigation.

Nevertheless, evidence of the superiority of surgical over conservative management is not evident (Collins 1983, 1984, Geisler *et al.* 1966).

A well-controlled randomized study comparing the various treatment regimes has never been done. Furthermore, variation in treatment plans, makes statistical analysis very difficult (Norrell 1979). This lack of statistical data undoubtedly contributes to the current dilemma regarding the optimal treatment of spinal injuries (Young *et al.* 1981).

## 2. Elements of Treatment

### *2.1. Clinical and Neuroradiological Data*

#### 2.1.1. Clinical Data

Technical features are closely related to the level of the fracture. At the thoracic level, fractures are more serious because of the increased vulnerability of the spinal cord due both to the poor arterial supply and to the relative narrowness of the thoracic canal compared to the lumbar canal (Dohn 1979, Hardy 1965). At the thoraco-lumbar junction and at lumbar level, the pathology can result in both conus and cauda equina lesions.

An accurate clinical evaluation is necessary to appreciate the prognosis and neurological recovery. This requires a careful and repeated study of motor and sensory function, the reflexes and the sphincters. Frankel *et al.* (1969) propose an evaluation in 5 stages:

(A) Complete: The lesion is complete both motor and sensory below the segmental level.

(B) Sensory only: Some sensation is present below the level of the lesion, but motor paralysis is complete.

(C) Motor useless: Some motor power is present below the lesion, but of no practical use.

(D) Motor useful: Useful motor power below the level of the lesion.

(E) Intact: Free of neurological symptoms.

Larson (1979), Larson *et al.* (1976), for evaluation assign the patients with incomplete lesions to functional categories A to G as follows:

(A) Walking without assistance, normal micturition.

(B) Walking with assistance, normal micturition.

(C) Walking without assistance, abnormal micturition.

(D) Walking with assistance, abnormal micturition.

(E) Unable to walk, some motor and sensory function, normal micturition.

(F) Unable to walk, some motor and sensory function, abnormal micturition.

(G) Paraplegic, sensory perception only, abnormal micturition.

Jelsma *et al.* (1982) propose the grading system of Chehrazi *et al.* (1981) with modification for the thora-columbar level. It is a method of quantitating neurological function numerically with a motor score (0 to 5), a sensory score (0 to 5). A total score of neurological function between 0 and 10 is obtained by adding the motor and sensory scores. In addition, in order to evaluate and compare recovery, they divide neurological injuries into the individually components related to the cauda equina or the conus medullaris.

Finally, the electrical study of somato-sensory evoked potentials helps greatly in all thoraco-lumbar lesions with neurological involvement (Cusick *et al.* 1979, Larson *et al.* 1966). This evaluation can be carried out before, during and after surgery. Schmidek *et al.* (1980) report that intra-operative studies help to prevent an increase in the patient's neural deficit during operation.

### 2.1.2. Neurological Data

Routine radiological studies of the spine includes plain X-rays and polytomography. Nowadays, the CT scan is the method of choice to thoroughly evaluate thoraco-lumbar spine fractures (Brant-Zawadzki *et al.* 1981, 1982). A CT scan allows optimal evaluation of the vertebral bodies, posterior elements and dimensions of the spinal canal pre- and postoperatively (Colley *et al.* 1978, Durward *et al.* 1981, Naidich *et al.* 1979).

CT scans will define precisely neural compression by a retropulsed bone fragment inside the spinal canal (Jelsma *et al.* 1982).

According to Schmidek *et al.* (1980), the best appreciation of the extent of the bony injury and deformity is obtained by CT scanning of the fracture site, which reveals an almost stereotyped group of findings: destruction of the body of the vertebra, retropulsion of a portion of the body into the spinal canal, solitary fracture of a pedicle, fracture of one or both laminae. These findings may be associated with dislocation and sagittal rotation of one vertebra on another.

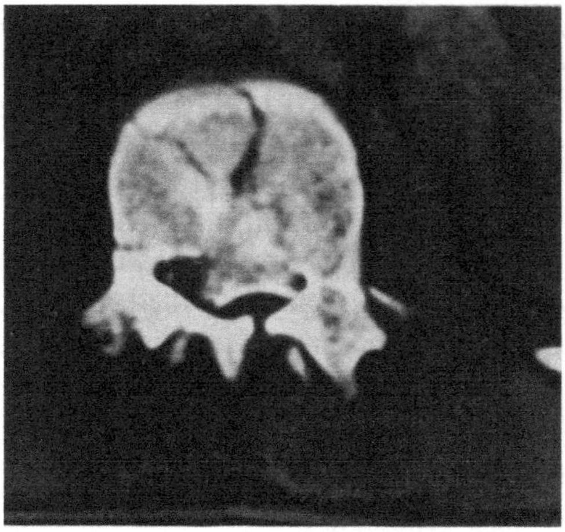

Fig. 1. CT scan showing a bursting fracture of L 1 vertebra with a retropulsed bone fragment causing canal compromise

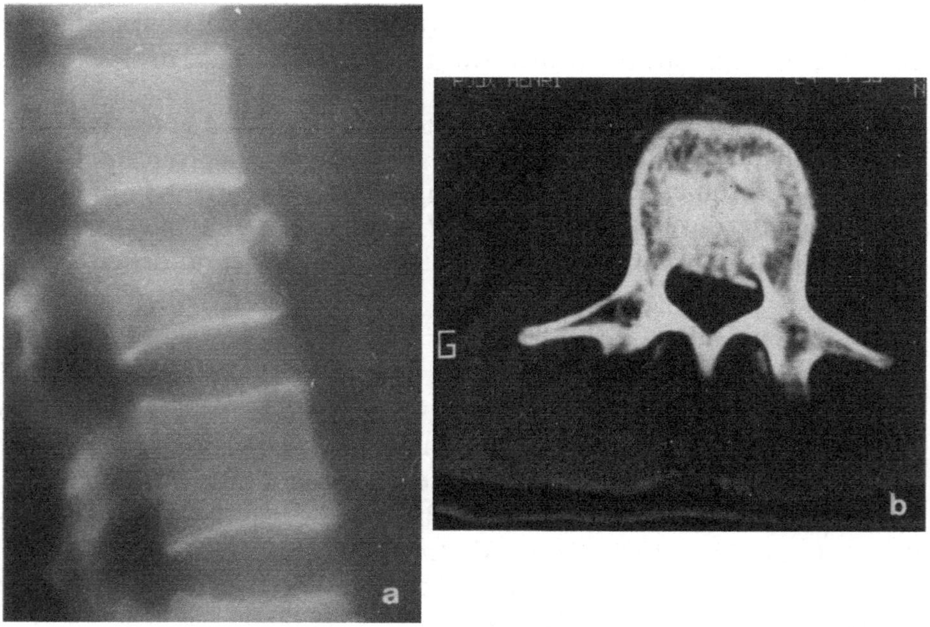


Fig. 2. Tomographic and CT scan views showing a L 2 wedge fracture with a retropulsed bone fragment in spinal canal from posterior and superior part of the vertebra

Durward *et al.* (1981) found a poor correlation between the degree of canal compromise measured by the CT scanner and the resulting neurological deficit. There are reasons for this; one is that in injuries where rotation and dislocation occurs, shearing and stretching forces, not compression, are the major factors in the production of the neurological lesion. We feel that the rate and degree of recovery is not related to the degree of canal decompression achieved at operation. There is a risk of delayed neural compression in the situation where there is a significantly narrowed spinal canal and no neurological signs, and there could be an indication for surgical intervention (Jelsma *et al.* 1982) (Fig. 1).

CT scanning may be completed by injection of a water-soluble intrathecal contrast medium which can quantify the degree of neural compression and may detect the presence of a dural rent (Brant-Zawadzki *et al.* 1982).

The CT scan data are usually sufficient to avoid routine preoperative myelography. A very interesting point is the comparison between the data from tomographic studies and the CT scan. This usually confirms that a retropulsed bone fragment or fragments in the spinal canal arise from the postero-superior part of the vertebral body and are wrenched away by the posterior common ligament (Fig. 2).

Indirect (closed) surgical reduction of the fracture often leaves behind the retropulsed bone fragment, which may only be removed by direct surgery. Also, it appears necessary after reduction, to check by either a CT scan or by myelography to see if a postero-superior retropulsed bone fragment is still present or not (Fig. 3).

Myelography with either iophendylate or metrizamide is reserved for two circumstance (Jelsma *et al.* 1982, Rogers *et al.* 1980, Schmidek *et al.* 1980):

(a) When the spinal column studies by plain X-rays, tomography and CT scanning did not seem to offer an adequate explanation for the neurological deficit. A contrast myelogram will show the presence of an extradural hematoma, an arachnoid cyst, or a herniated disc, but will give little information about the state of the spinal cord, indeed, a spinal block can be attributed to either spinal cord laceration or from cord edema.

(b) Intra-operatively after reduction of the spine or of bone removal, to confirm the adequacy of the decompression of neural structures.

Spinal cord angiography has been advocated to evaluate thoraco-lumbar fractures with neural involvement to identify the artery of Adamkiewicz, to demonstrate any displacement and to show the site of its origin, and thereby during a surgical approach, to avoid injury to it and the risk of cord ischemia (Bussat *et al.* 1973, Paul *et al.* 1975).

It is likely that in the future I.R.M. will permit studies and controls for thoraco-lumbar spine injuries, both pre- and postoperatively.

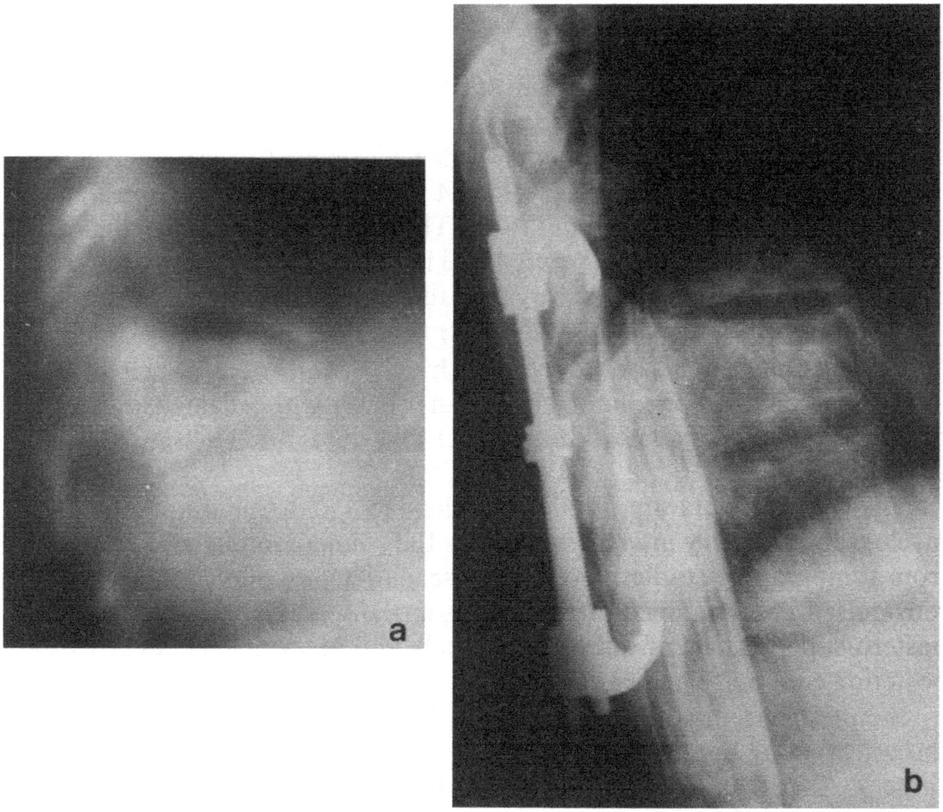

Fig. 3. Postoperative myelography in wedge fracture of T 11. Control of the posterior wall of the vertebra and the cavity of the spinal canal

### *2.2. Anatomical and Functional Data*

#### 2.2.1. The Fracture and Its Mechanism

It has been emphasized that spinal stability depends upon the integrity of either the anterior column (vertebral bodies and discs) or the posterior column (apophyseal joints) (Davis 1938, Lafferty *et al.* 1977, Petter 1933, Roaf 1960).

The plane of the facets plays an important role in determining the nature of the fracture as it relates to the mechanism of injury.

Three regions can be identified. Throughout the thoracic spine to the T 11–T 12 articulation, the plane of the facets is close to the coronal plane of the body. The costotransverse and costovertebral articulations may stabilize this region to some extent, but the plane of these facets permits flexion, extension, tilt, and rotation. The strong apophyseal joints overlap markedly, and tend to hold in flexion stresses such a trauma, whereas the weaker vertebral body collapses.

The thoracolumbar junction presents a different problem. The most common mechanism of injury is hyperflexion. After the cervical spine, the thoracolumbar junction is the most mobile and vulnerable region of the spinal column. 40% of all spinal cord injuries occur at this level (Kaufer *et al.* 1966). The T 12–L 1 articulation differs strikingly from that of T 11–T 12 in that the inferior facets lie near the sagittal plane. The T 12–L 1 articulation is the first and weakest of the sagittal articulations. It permits either a compression fracture in flexion, or less often, an impaction fracture in which the mechanism is extension (Miller *et al.* 1980).

In the lumbar regions, the facets are also in the sagittal plane.

Böhler describes a classification of fractures resulting from flexion into 5 groups. He emphasizes their frequency and on the association of vertebral body damage with posterior lesions. Watson-Jones (1938, 1949, 1958) describes three kinds of lesions:

(a) Fractures of spinous and transverse processes.

(b) Fractures of parts of the vertebral body which receive and convey the weight of body.

(c) Facet fractures which alter the continuity of the neural canal and of spinal cord integrity.

Concerning vertebral body fractures, he recognizes three classical lesions:

(a) The wedge fracture resulting from axial compression of the spine in slight flexion.

(b) The burst fracture in relation to sudden impact of the antero-inferior corner of superior vertebral body into the inferior vertebral body during an acute flexion.

(c) Fracture-dislocation connected with a predominant active horizontal force. In this case, there are lesions of the posterior elements in the form of luxation or fracture of an articular process.

According to Watson-Jones (1949, 1958), wedge fractures and burst fractures are stable, and fracture-dislocations are unstable.

Nicoll (1949, 1962) states that burst fractures are associated with severe axial loadings and describes a peculiar anatomical lesion: the fracture with a lateral compression, and a new mechanism, of rotation. He believes that lesions of the posterior elements are due to a flexion-rotation force and that fractures of the pedicles are very infrequent and more often accompany severe dislocation-fractures.

Holdsworth (1963, 1970) and Pennal (1966) confirm the axial character of the forces in burst fractures and explain that the vertebral body bursts under the impact of the nucleus.

Holdsworth (1963) describes 4 mechanisms: flexion, flexion-rotation, extension and compression. Like Nicoll (1949), he believes that rotation forces are in the main responsible for fractures of the neural arch, the posterior articular process and the posterior ligaments. Kaufer and Hayes (1966) distinguish five varieties of fracture-dislocations according to the bony lesions associated with luxation:

Type 1: Isolated luxation.

Type 2: Luxation with wedge fracture of the inferior vertebral body.

Type 3: Articular luxation and vertebral body fracture with sliding of fragments.

Type 4: Unilateral articular luxation.

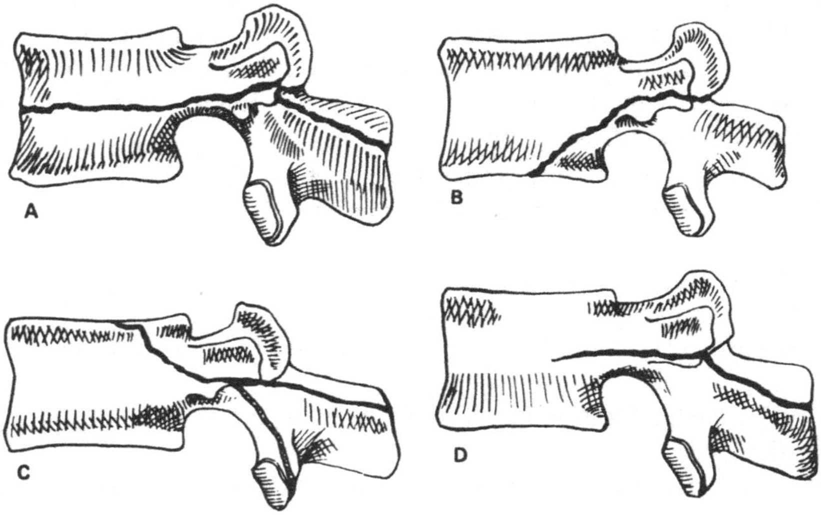


Fig. 4. Classification of Chance's fractures proposed by Fuentes *et al.* (1984)

Type 5: Fracture of both articular processes.

Chance (1948) describes a special lesion, where there is disruption of the vertebral body by horizontal splitting of this formation and the neural arches through the pedicles, with a minimal decrease in the anterior height of the involved vertebral body and without forward or lateral displacement of the superior vertebra. The site is usually between the first and third lumbar vertebra. The spinal canal is rarely threatened. This fracture is induced by a mechanism of flexion-distraction (Grantham *et al.* 1976, Rennie and Mitchell 1973) and the mechanism can be related to a "seat-belt" fracture (Smith *et al.* 1969).

Fuentes *et al.* (1984) propose the following classification (Fig. 4):

Type 1: The line involves the whole vertebra (posterior arch and body) in a horizontal manner. The fracture is unstable.

Type 2: The line continues into the posterior and inferior third of the vertebral body. The fracture is unstable.

Type 3: The line continues into the posterior and superior third. The fracture is unstable.

Type 4: The line is incomplete and disappears in the posterior third of the vertebral body (the fracture is stable).

Miller *et al.* (1980) describe an unstable lumbar spine fracture, "the impaction fracture", characterized in antero-posterior X-rays views by separation of the pedicular shadows. This lesion is often associated with posterior interlaminar herniation of the cauda equina through a dorsal dural tear and antero-lateral entrapment or amputation of the nerve root. According to Jelsma *et al.* (1982) an "impaction" fracture is a severe burst fracture.

Roaf (1960) concludes that compressive forces are chiefly absorbed by the vertebral body, resulting in fracture, and that rotational injury is the most common cause of posterior ligamentous disruption.

Kelly and Whitesides (1968) observe that the anterior column structures of the spine, the vertebral bodies, are under compressive loads, and that the posterior structures, the ligamentous complex, are under tensile loads. An understanding of this concept is basic to determine the kind of lesions and to choose a suitable form of internal fixation.

Jacobs *et al.* (1980) divide their cases into biomechanical types and describe:

(a) Distraction and flexion-distraction injuries.

(b) Burst fractures (including compression fracture of the anterior vertebral body).

(c) Fracture-dislocations.

A rotational instability may be a component of any of the previously described injuries if the facet joints are fractured or if there is significant translational deformity of the anterior structures, and thus fracture-dislocations are nearly always rotationally unstable. This biomechanical approach analyzes the force applied to the spine and determines the structures that have failed and consequently the best treatment for immediate and permanent stabilization.

### 2.2.2. The Concept of Stability or Instability

The studies by Nicoll (1949) and Watson-Jones (1949) will be discussed in detail below.

Watson-Jones (1949) pays particular attention to the inter and supraspinous ligaments and to the articular processes. Nicoll (1949) like Mallet-Guy (1938) and Schmorl (1956) particularly stress lesions of the intervertebral disc. Holdsworth (1963) notes the important role of the articular processes and the posterior ligamentous complex. Nicoll (1949) describes:

(a) Stable fractures with anterior and lateral wedge and fractures of neural arch, above L 4.

(b) Unstable fracture including subluxations with disruption of the inter spinous ligament, i.e., a severe anterior wedge—burst fractures—fracture-dislocations and fractures of the neural arch of L 4 and L 5.

Decoulx *et al.* (1958, 1959) and Rieunaud (1970) attribute spinal stability to the integrity of the "posterior wall", formed by the posterior part of the vertebral body, the posterior aspects of the discs, and the common posterior vertebral ligament.

Roy-Camille (1970) mentions the "Middle vertebral segment", i.e., the part constituted by the "posterior wall", the pedicles and the superior and inferior articular processes.

Louis (1974, 1977) proposes an anatomical description of the thoraco-lumbar spine:

(a) Ventrally, an anterior column, made by the stacking up of vertebral bodies and intervertebral discs. This complex is resistant to axial loadings.

(b) Dorsally the two posterior columns of articular processes, which are resistant to antero-posterior tensions.

(c) The junction between these 3 columns is formed by horizontal bony bridges (pedicles and laminae). There are horizontal elements on which the ligaments are inserted and muscles are inserted on to the spinous and transverse processes. These lesions of the anterior column and lesions of the elements on which ligaments and muscles are inserted determine possible "vertical" instability. Lesions of posterior articular columns are responsible for "horizontal" instability. Injuries of the junction between the 3 columns will increase the instability resulting from other lesions. A "mixed" instability associates a "vertical" instability with a "horizontal" instability.

Louis (1977) distinguishes the prodominant bony instability, which is of good evolution, because it heals soundly and the predominant discal or ligamentous instability which has a bad prognosis, because it does not do so. He notes that a bony defect of the spine is more serious than a simple linear fracture.

The body defect usually appears in two circumstances relevant to therapy: (a) the reduction of a significant traumatic kyphosis over 25°, by a wedge fracture, causes the emergence of lacunae in the disengaged space, and (b) laminectomy produces a posterior defect which impairs the posterior stresses and consequently the factors for stabilization.

There are three categories in the report by Roberts *et al.* (1970): (a) wedge compression, (b) compression burst, and (c) rotational fracture-dislocation. The spine in patients in the first and last groups rarely fuse spontaneously and there is a high incidence of instability.

Jelsma *et al.* (1982) diagnose instability preoperatively, when there is a dislocation, a severe burst fracture, or a wedge fracture with marked subluxation, traumatic spondylolisthesis, or horizontally fractured pedicles, i.e., chance fracture. They do not consider increasing angulation or increasing compression of a vertebral body to be indications of instability.

Seljeskog (1982) considers that major compression injuries involving more than 50% of the height of the ventral part of the body should be considered to be potentially unstable. If the posterior elements are not involved, he manages such patients monoperatively, but has recourse to surgery when the posterior elements are involved or when a progressive kyphosis appears.

Instability is obvious to Schmidek *et al.* (1980) when a comminution of the vertebral body is present, a sagittal rotation of one vertebral body on another by 2.5 mm, a sharply wedged (50%) compression of the body of the vertebra, or dislocation greater than 2 mm.

Jacobs *et al.* (1980) have a very extensive concept of instability. Any injury of the thoraco-lumbar spine sufficiently severe to be associated with a neurological deficit is assumed to be mechanically unsound for early ambulatory treatment without internal fixation. Secondly, injuries that may result in neurological damage are also considered to be unstable. Their third indication is an injury that may lead to "chronic instability", and late neurological deficit by progressive deformity. The so-called stable compression fracture is frequently placed in this category (Nash *et al.* 1977).

In conclusion, it is necessary to recognize that the classification of these injuries and the definition of stability has not been precisely defined.

## 3. Methods of Treatment

### *3.1. The Methods of Treatment Concerning Osteo-articular Lesions*

#### 3.1.1. Orthopedic Methods

The aim of orthopedic surgeons is to reduce and immobilize the fracture. The technique of reduction between two tables described by Watson-Jones (1958) is noted but especially the famous work of Böhler (1944) with the method of reduction in hyperlordosis, followed by a plaster body jacket in a position of reduction and by active reeducation, which for some physicians, represented the only treatment. This treatment was recommended by Magnus (1929) and Nicoll (1949) for stable fractures. Nicoll (1949) found that anatomical reduction is not necessary for a good functional result. For stable fractures, he advocated three to four weeks of bed rest. For unstable fractures without neurological deficit, he found that a protective plaster in the position of deformity resulted in spontaneous anterior fusion with a better functional result than is obtained by surgical fusion. In unstable fractures with paraplegia, he observed that any hope of cord or root recovery required open or closed reduction and the maintenance demanded grafting or internal fixation.

The technique of Böhler (1944) remains the basis of orthopedic treatment methods to date.

Modern reduction (Louis 1975) is possible using the apparatus for reduction for scoliosis, without anesthesia, and under radiographic control. The interest of this method of reduction is that it permits various handling in all planes with great accuracy in the intensity and the direction of strengths.

The patient is placed in a dorsal decubitus position with supports under the neck and the buttocks.

An axial traction is set up with a cephalic sling and pelvic traction. A dynamometer allows the surgeon to control the force of traction. A broad webbing band placed under the spinous process of the injured zone, can provide the hyperlordosis manoeuvre. Under radiological control, axial traction is carried out until the posterior aspect of the vertebral body has recovered a relative height. The lordosis manoeuvre is discontinued when the anterior wedge is corrected and when the vertebral plates became parallel. Wedge fractures and burst fractures require a pull of about 5 to 15 kilogrammes, dislocation-fractures about 15 to 25 kilogrammes. Reduction is followed by applying a padded plaster body jacket. The body jacket requires three areas of support: sternal, pelvic and thoraco-lumbar. For upper thoracic lesions, a chin support may be a useful addition.

A patient with no neurological abnormalities may be permitted up some hours later. Daily physiotherapy is required including static contractions of the trunk muscles. The plaster is removed after the third month. Regular, radiological controls are made. The treatment is equally possible with moulded plastic which is lighter, but may be less rigid.

Reduction made in emergency situations can restore the normal anatomical alignment and thus allow decompression of nervous structures. A delayed surgical procedure can be performed if required. It could be argued, also, that halo-traction should be expected to provide sufficient realignment to obviate the need for an immediate operation. Between orthopedic and neurosurgical procedures, stabilization is still possible by exoskeletal spinal procedures.

## 3.1.2. Surgical Methods

### 3.1.2 (a) Surgical Approaches

#### i Posterior Approaches

The classical posterior approach remains the standard neurosurgical procedure for a laminectomy, to explore the spinal canal to repare a dural injury, or to remove a posterior compressive element. It also permits realignment or stabilization of a fracture, with or without laminectomy (Bradford *et al.* 1977). This approach may be used alone or be combined by some other surgical procedure.

The enlarged posterior approach (postero-lateral approach), described by Carson *et al.* (1971), and by Menard (1894), with a costotransversectomy, may be employed for the removal of a thoracic disc protrusion and for the drainage of a tuberculous paraspinal abscess in Pott's paraplegia. This approach was advocated for thoraco-lumbar spine fractures with the object of a combined decompression of neural elements and stabilization of the spine. Using rongeurs or an air drill, the lateral part of the laminae, the articular processes, and one or more pedicles, are removed at the level which will permit lateral exposure of the area of spinal deformity. The nerve roots are identified and the lateral dural sac is clearly exposed at the fracture site. If there are any obvious pieces of loose bone and disc fragments within the canal, they are removed. More often, the anterior deformity is due to a retropulsed portion of vertebral body and the technique permits decompression without the need for retraction of the dura and the spinal cord (Erickson 1978, Erickson *et al.* 1977, Flesch *et al.* 1977, Jelsma *et al.* 1982, Schmidek *et al.* 1980). The major deficiencies of this operation are the limited exposure and the difficulties in finding normal anatomical landmarks.

ii Anterior approaches include the transpleural at the thoracic level, or transperitoneal for the anterior lumbo-sacral area and at L 4 and L 5. These approaches are seldom used and present difficult technical problems concerning the prevertebral nerves and vessels and the peritoneum, especially at the L 4 and L 5 levels.

Of more interest is the anterior extraperitoneal approach described by Cid Dos Santos for sympathectomy. This is an approach carried out with the patient in a dorsal decubitus position, which permits wide access to the vertebral bodies of L 3 and L 4.

Lesoin *et al.* (1984) report an antero-internal approach for the whole lumbar spine by modifying the incision proposed by Cid Dos Santos.

iii Lateral Approaches

The postero-lateral approach involves the resection of a sufficient portion of one or two ribs to allow the development of a truly lateral extrapleural exposure of the spine. It has been suggested by Capener (1954) for traumatic cases when there is anterior cord compression. Chou (1978) and Larson *et al.* (1976) have also described this technique.

In the thoracic region the approach is extrapleural. It is usually necessary to resect at least two ribs, the corresponding transverse process, pedicles and the apophyseal joints to provide full visualization. In the lumbar region, the approach is extraperitoneal and the plane of dissection lies between the erector spinae muscles and the quadratus lumborum.

In the experience of Larson *et al.* (1976), concerning 62 patients operated by this method, the highest vertebral level approached was T 3, and the lowest S 1; 60% were between T 9 and L 2.

The antero-lateral approach although requiring a thoracotomy, provides extensive exposure of vertebral bodies. Developed for the treatment of Pott's paraplegia, the procedure was first reported by Hodgson (1956) and has been advocated for the treatment of trauma involving the anterior elements of the spine. It necessitates a cutaneous incision centered over the tenth and eleventh ribs and is performed with the patient in the lateral decubitus position (Young *et al.* 1981). The spine is approached through the retroperitoneal and retropleural spaces and there is an easy exposure of the anterolateral surfaces of the bodies of T 11 to L 2 vertebrae.

Louis (1982) modified the Hodgson procedure, and performs the operation with the patient in a dorsal decubitus position. An incision centered over the ninth rib allows a perfect exposure of the thoraco-lumbar junction with the patient on axial traction and in a hyperlordosis position.

iv Mixed approaches, these include two operative procedures: posterior and anterior (Louis 1974, Yocum *et al.* 1970). Either procedure is carried out initially or with the two surgical procedures being separated by 15 days (Chabannes *et al.* 1982).

### 3.1.2 (b) Techniques of Reduction and Stabilization

i Posterior osteosynthesis by metal plates screwed into the vertebral pedicles and the articular processes. This technique of osteosynthesis was first described by Roy-Camille *et al.* (1970, 1973, 1977) and precised by the work of Gonon *et al.* (1974) and Saillant (1976). Two plates, 10 mm wide, 4 mm thick, with holes spaced at 13 mm intervals are used. The spacing of the holes corresponds to the average spacing between the pedicles and the articular processes. The holes for pediculo-corporeal screws are 4.8 mm in diameter and corresponding screws are 4.5 mm in diameter. The holes for the articular process are smaller (3.8 mm), also the screws (3.5 mm). The length of the screws is 14 to 15 mm for the articular process; 35 to 40 mm for pedicles. The plates seen in profile, are curved to conform to the normal lumbar lordosis and are malleable, so that their curve may be changed.

Plates with 4, 5, 7, 9, 11, and 15 holes are available. The length of the plate chosen depends on the length of the posterior arthrodesis desired, in such a way that each extreme pedicle is opposite to a hole in the plate. The point of penetration of the screw, at the thoracic and lumbar levels, is made at the lower edge of the articulation. In the lumbar area, the articular surfaces are in a sagittal plane and the point of entry is 1 mm inferior to the lower edge of the joint.

In the thoracic area, the articulatory (joint) space is in a frontal plane, hidden by the inferior articular process. The point of entry in this situation, will be 1 mm under the lower edge of the lower articular process. Drilling for insertion of the screw must be done perpendicular to the vertebra in a strictly symmetrical plane. The length of arthrodesis is variable (Roy-Camille *et al.* 1977) fixing the two vertebrae immediately above and below the injured level, in those with corporeal lesions, and in patients with an

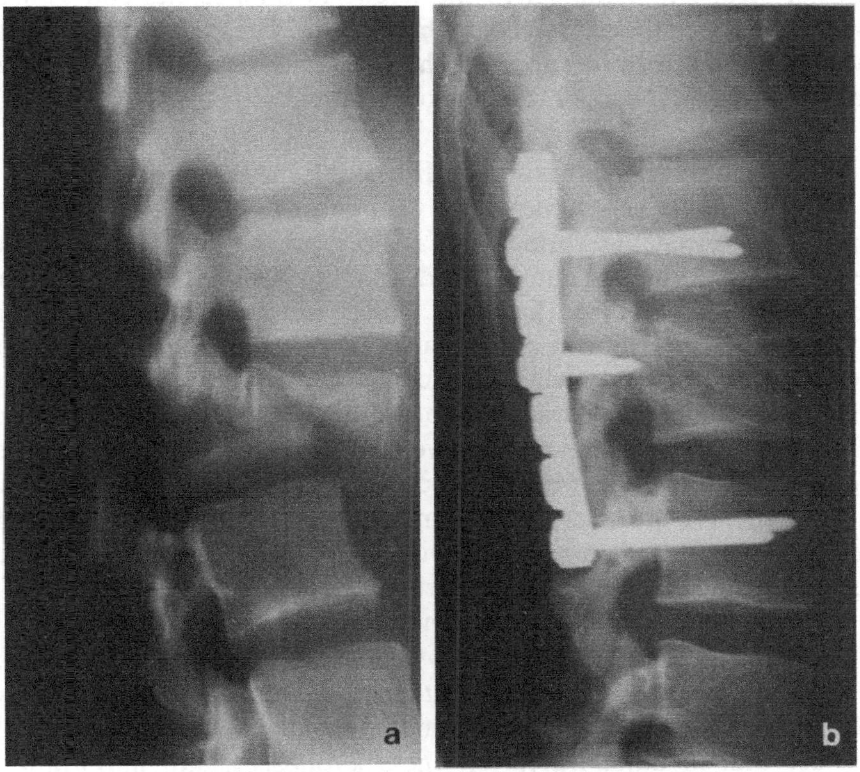


Fig. 5. Complex fracture of L 2. Fixation with Roy-Camille's plates

isolated dislocation. Screwing the pedicles is difficult because of anatomical changes, and peroperative identification of the pedicles, by a lateral X-ray, is useful. When the screws are tightened, the curve of the plate produces excellent reduction of bony deformations. The osteosynthesis is strong, stable and permits early mobilization, the day after the operation, without the necessity for a plaster corset. It eliminates the problems of secondary displacement, compression or accentuation of kyphosis. It also permits rapid normal physical activity (Fig. 5).

The lateral position of the plates may permit a laminectomy procedure. Occasionally, especially, in the lower regions of the spine where the stresses are greatest, some screws break after mobilization of the patient, but without any effect on bony fusion. This surgical technique has been adopted by many authors for thoraco-lumbar fractures (Brunon *et al.* 1973, Hermann 1979, Lagarrigues *et al.* 1980). Some authors have modified the plates (Vlahovitch *et al.* 1977), others have modified the method of insertion of the screws into the pedicles, especially for the lower lumbar vertebrae (Fuentes *et al.* 1984). Unlike Roy-Camille, Lesoin *et al.* (1982), never use articular screws to complement the screws in the pedicles and they also insert a screw into the damaged vertebra (Fig. 6). The tolerance of the plates is very good. If discomfort appears, the plates can be removed after about a year, when bony consolidation has occurred.

ii Posterior osteosynthesis with distraction instrumentation

The Harrington instrumentation (Harrington 1967, 1973) is used by applying two mechanical principles: (a) direct pressure of the rod applied at the apex of the kyphosis, and (b) the distracting device produces tension on the anterior longitudinal ligament which restores normal height and provides normal alignment of the fractured vertebra. Care is taken not to over-distract. The instrumentation includes two rods notched at their upper parts. Two superior distraction hooks are placed under the articular processes of the superior vertebra two interspaces above the fracture level and two inferior hooks are placed on the inferior lamina at the second interspace below the fracture. Two intact vertebrae above and two below the fracture must be spanned to provide a lever arm long enough to reduce the fracture and to maintain the reduction. The distraction hooks are placed in the same manner as for the treatment of scoliosis.

This technique is used by many Anglo-Saxon authors (Bradford *et al.* 1977, Convery *et al.* 1978, Dickson *et al.* 1978, Durward *et al.* 1981, Jelsma *et al.* 1982, Katznelson 1969, Schmidek *et al.* 1980). Perves *et al.* 1973 consider that in burst fractures, where kyphosis is not important, the Harrington technique which restores the height of vertebrae is suitable.

Jelsma *et al.* (1982) use the method to correct the angulation and anterior wedging of the vertebral body in wedge fractures, to reduce burst fractures until the normal distance between the vertebrae above and below the fracture is restored, and also to reduce dislocations. For Flesch *et al.* (1977), the technique has been adapted for dislocation-fractures and burst fractures.

Durward *et al.* (1981) state that in patients where the bony spinal canal is compromised with suspected neural compression from retropulsed bone fragments, Harrington distraction does not result in reduction of the retropulsed bone and consequently, to achieve decompression in such patients it is necessary to surgically remove the vertebral body and the bone fragments.

Jacobs *et al.* (1980) recommend that burst fractures, wedge fractures and

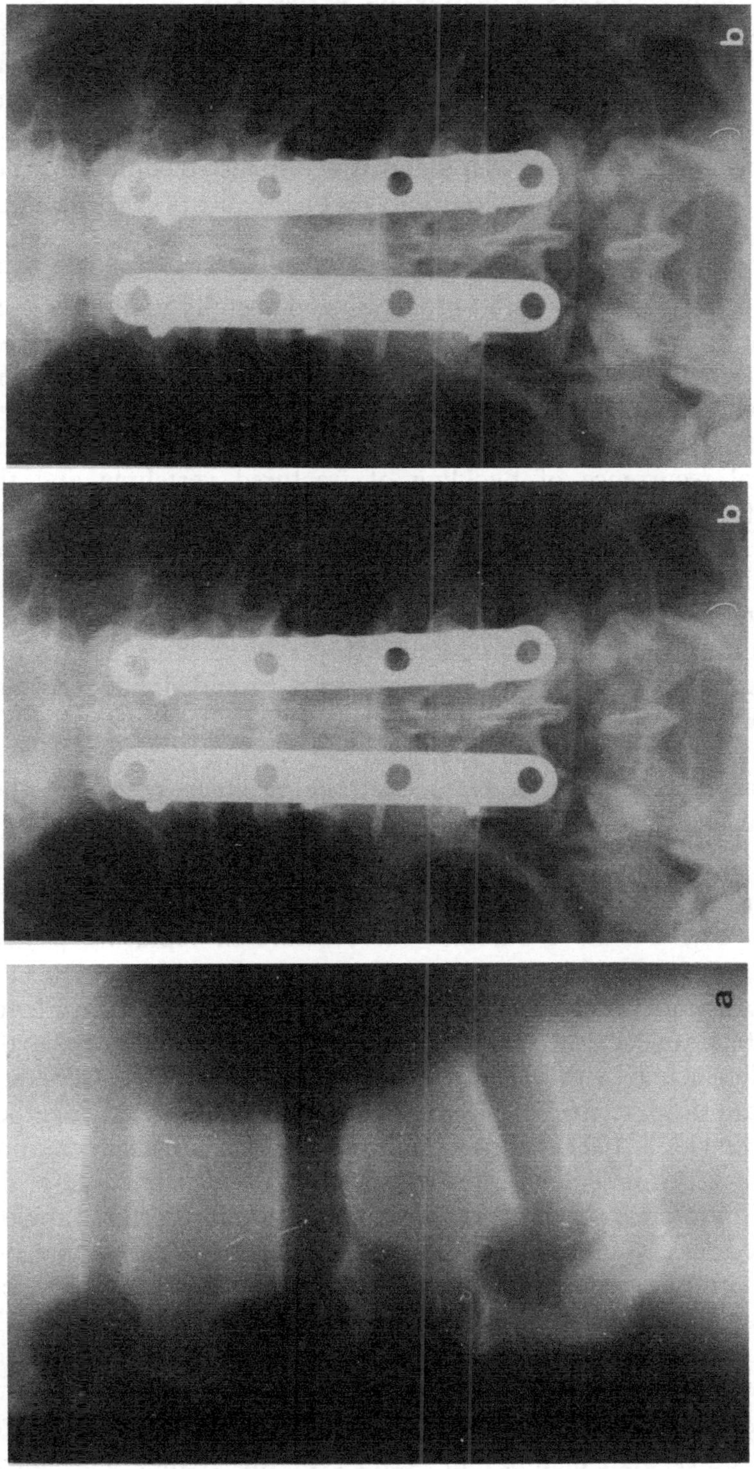


Fig. 6. Chance's fracture. Reduction and fixation with Roy-Camille's plates. Screws are inserted into the vertebrae above and below the fracture and also in the damaged vertebra

fracture dislocations require a distracting device. The disadvantage of distraction rods is that they necessitate a larger exposure and immobilize a much longer spinal segment. Beattie (1969) uses a similar apparatus as Harrington: the Knodt distraction rods, which immobilizes only three vertebrae.

Lagarrigues *et al.* (1980) consider that distraction instrumentation is not well adapted to the stabilization of the bony lesion because of the distraction effect. They only use the technique during surgery as a means of reduction.

Recently Fountain *et al.* (1978) reported on the complications with Harrington rod treatment: pain, progressive deformity, failure of instrumentation, infection, alignment without reduction. For Jacobs *et al.* (1980) the mechanical problems of progressive deformity and alignment without decompression suggest a failure to follow biomechanical principles. Michel *et al.* (1976) also note the anatomical failure of the technique because of the partial recurrence of buckling of fractured vertebrae and the recurrence of global kyphosis.

With the Harrington rod procedure, some authors recommend control by mylography either during or after surgery to demonstrate the effectiveness of decompression (Jelsma *et al.* 1982, Young *et al.* 1981).

The mobilization of a patient after such surgery is variable, usually one to two weeks after surgery, with or without a moulded body cast or removable plastic body jacket (Convery *et al.* 1978, Dickson *et al.* 1978, Erickson *et al.* 1977, Jelsma *et al.* 1982).

It is possible retain the rods unless they produce pain or other complications (Jelsma *et al.* 1982).

iii Posterior osteosynthesis with compression instrumentation:

Here, the objective is to stabilize the fracture in replacing passive ligamentous structures and active muscular structures destroyed by the injury, while the anterior bony elements withstand the compressive loads (Fig. 7). The fixation occurs in lordosis. The compression system utilizes the tension band principle, with bone carrying the anterior compressive stress and the implant the posterior tensile stress. This method has been described by Kempf *et al.* (1973, 1977) and is similar to Harrington instrumentation used in the surgery for scoliosis. Hooks are placed on the laminae of the superior and the inferior vertebrae in relation to the injured vertebra and the rods are placed on each side of the midline. The apparatus is very strong, but it requires anterior bony integrity, indeed, compression may cause displacement of discal or bony elements into the spinal canal. Perves *et al.* (1973) prefer this technique in dislocation-fractures and wedge fractures because of the lordosis effect.

Convery *et al.* (1978) favour compression instrumentation in fracture-dislocations rather than distraction, because of the greater mechanical stability and because distraction performed in other sites usually delays bony union.

Flesch *et al.* (1977) employ the Harrington distraction system for fracture-dislocations and burst fractures in which controlled corrective forces are needed, and use compression system for fractures producing an

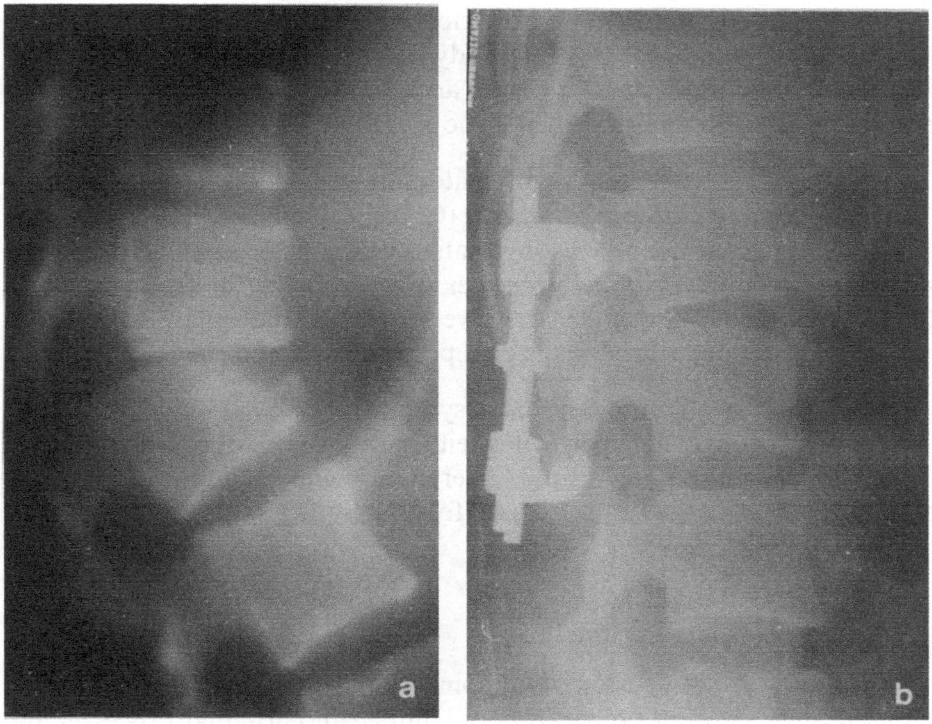

Fig. 7. Dislocation at T 12–L 1 level, with only ligamentous disruption. Compression fixation with Knodt instrumentation

unstable kyphosis, and for Chance type fractures in which posterior compression is needed for stability. Fuentes *et al.* (1984) suggest compression device in Chance type fracture, type I, in which the fracture involves the whole vertebra, in a horizontal manner.

Jacobs *et al.* (1980) report that these distraction and flexion injuries, in which there is a predominant posterior ligamentous disruption respond well to compression fixation. Patients with complete destruction of a vertebral body and permanent total paraplegia are amenable to a compression device, because it is not necessary to reconstruct the normal anatomy if the neurological structures are destroyed. Moreover, the shorter length of the spine immobilized by a compression system compared to the length when distraction rods are used is a distinct advantage in the rehabilitation of the paraplegic patient.

Vlahovitch *et al.* (1978) report the treatment of fractures and dislocations of the lower lumbar vertebrae with Kempf's material. We are impressed with the follow-up and the stability of the fixation and recommend the method for all unstable lesions of the lower lumbar vertebrae. The Kempf's material is very well adapted to lower lumbar region, because it restores the posterior tensile stresses and respects the lumbar curve, but, a posterior interbody fusion is needed to stabilize discal injuries and important burst fractures and avoid displacements of discal or bony fragments compressing nerve roots.

iv Posterior osteosynthesis with plates screwed on to spinous processes:

This technique has been little used (Creyssel 1950, Delcoux *et al.* 1955) and necessitates the use of Wilson's plates (1952). These are placed on each side of two or three spinous processes to immobilize the fractured area. Insertion and removal to the plates is very easy, but the apparatus is strong only if an anterior arthrodesis is also performed (Louis *et al.* 1975).

v Anterior or antero-lateral osteosynthesis:

This procedure can be performed either with plates only, or associated with an anterior interbody fusion. Other instruments used for the treatment of scoliosis, may in the future be used for traumatic lesions, such as Dwyer instrumentation (1969).

### 3.1.2 (c) Bony Spine Fusions

The place for bony fusion of the spine is now discussed. This is achieved either posteriorly after preparation of laminae and articular processes and an interbody bony fusion in the manner of Cloward (1963) or by an anterior interbody procedure. Autogenous bone such as iliac, tibial, peroneal or ribs may be used. In the future, heterogeneous preserved bone will be available.

Usually used in association with instrumentation, bony fusion is sometimes difficult to achieve.

For recent fractures, Roy-Camille *et al.* (1970) propose instrumentation without a bone graft; similarly Lesoin *et al.* (1981) do not combine bone grafts and Roy-Camille's plates.

Dickson *et al.* (1978) advocate Harrington instrumentation and bony fusion of fracture-dislocations of the spine. They generally fuse the entire area extending from the superior to the inferior distraction hooks in patients who have complete lesions, and fuse only across the fractured segment in patients with incomplete cord lesions.

Flesch *et al.* (1977) manage unstable fractures and fracture-dislocations with Harrington instrumentation either with distraction rods or compression rods and in all cases perform a postero-lateral fusion with autogenous iliac-bone grafts.

Jacobs *et al.* (1980) question the length of the rods and the indication for fusion. If the rods extend three levels above and three below the area of injury, they perform a bony fusion confined to the area of injury in patients with a fracture-dislocation and no fusion in the case of burst fractures, with good results. When they use the method with rods placed from two levels above to two levels below, with the fusion extending alone the length of the rods, their results are less good.

Convery *et al.* (1978) with the same instrumentation, stabilize the shortest segment possible and carry out a bony fusion. Terver (1975) has shown that after removal of Roy-Camille's plates, mobility of the fractured area is present in 26% of patients, and this is responsible for a progessive degree of kyphosis, testifying to the lack of consolidation. This occurs whatever the quality of osteosynthesis, and the duration of application of the apparatus (beyond two years) and even without a laminectomy.

These data suggest that a bone graft should be carried out, or do not remove the plates if they are well tolerated (Lagarrigues 1980). It is evident that instrumentation is only an indirect means which favours consolidation by immobilization of the fractured area.

Louis (1975) notes that orthopedic reduction of a wedge fracture results in a satisfactory radiological appearance, but after 3 months in a plaster corset, buckling may recur. His explanation is that a normal looking vertebral body has very important defects.

The consolidation is not accomplished under pressure, but under distraction because of the plaster corset and the reeducation in hyper-lordosis. Thus, the spongy spans are not adapted to the physiological stresses and collapse, due to flexion movements of the trunk.

The same, most probably applies to the use of wire to maintain reduction and stabilization. This also interests Chabannes *et al.* (1982).

In all these situations, bony spinal fusion seems to be required.

## *3.2. The Methods of Treatment Concerning Neurological Lesions*

### 3.2.1. Laminectomy

Spinal decompression by laminectomy was for a long time the surgical treatment of choice for thoraco-lumbar injuries with the object of exploring the injured area and decompressing the spinal cord. But the operation of laminectomy became a matter of great controversy, and has in some degree continued, but objections include the risk of aggravating the neurological status (Bennasy *et al.* 1967, Bohlman 1974, Carey 1965, Harris 1963, Guttmann 1949, 1973, Kaufer *et al.* 1966, Morgan *et al.* 1971), and also when laminectomy is the only surgical procedure, it mays lead to greater instability with increased spinal deformity (Dickson *et al.* 1973).

Another criticism is that thoraco-lumbar cord injuries usually cause an anterior cord lesion due to the posterior displacement of fragments of bone and intervertebral disc (Bradford *et al.* 1976, Paul *et al.* 1975, Pierce 1969, Schneider 1955), and that finally reduction of fractures may be an effective method of decompressing the spinal canal contents.

Laminectomy still has some support, and some definite indications. Houdart *et al.* (1973) state that it is useful at the lumbar level where the problem is one of radicular involvement.

Flesch *et al.* (1977) perform laminectomy in most of their patients with an incomplete lesion of the spinal cord, conus or cauda equina.

Seljeskog (1982) has been impressed with the inadequacy of the technique of blind fracture reduction utilizing the Harrington rod technique without decompression. In spite of reduction and realignment of the fracture, fragments and disc material can easily be left behind. In light of this, he carries out a lateral laminectomy to ensure complete decompression of the spinal canal. At the same time, the dura can be repaired and prolapsed nerve roots reduced. Harris (1977) stated the importance of clinical and myelographic recognition of dural and arachnoid tears and prolapse of cauda equina roots in certain patients with lumbar spine injuries, and the importance of early operative treatment for these patients; myelography and laminectomy being essential; the prolapsed nerve roots are replaced and the dura repaired.

For Lagarrigues *et al.* (1980) laminectomy facilitates the pedicular screwing of Roy-Camille's plates.

Lesoin *et al.* (1981) justifies laminectomy for several reasons. The lesion can be seen, and compression of the swollen cord relieved, and an aponeurotic graft is applied. It may permit removal of small fragments of bone that might eventually move and further injure the spinal cord. In 10 of their patients, laminectomy revealed an extradural hematoma or an arachnoid cyst.

Chabannes *et al.* (1982) considering the association of paraplegia and complex lesions of the vertebrae recommend a laminectomy before arthrodesis.

### 3.2.2. Medical Treatment

There are several animal spinal cord injuries studies where various forms of treatment appear to have been beneficial, these include therapy used against edema (corticosteroids, mannitol); or ischemia (Papaverine, local hypothermia, hyperbaric oxygen, longitudinal myelotomy) and the opium antagonist naxolone (Flamm *et al.* 1982). The basis for some of the therapies is related to the existence in the contused spinal cord of a significant increase in the levels of catecholamines, which are responsible for vasospasm and ischaemic posttraumatic phenomena. Thus, there is an interest in the use of anticatecholaminic drugs (tyroxine, reserpine, dopa), and for longitudinal myelotomy in an attempt to halt the release of catecholamines at the site of injury. Pettegrew *et al.* (1976) report on the use of myelotomy. Nevertheless, most surgeons are reluctant to incise a swollen spinal cord lest necrotic tissues spew forth, and it is very doubtful indeed that a delayed procedure can benefit the patient; success, in all cases, depends on acting promptly after an accident.

The effect of these different treatments is very difficult to determine in man.

Bricolo *et al.* (1976) have reported eight patients with acute spinal cord injury treated by local extradural cooling and have justified the application of this procedure by their encouraging results. But the procedure is not easy, a laminectomy is needed, and we have doubts about the procedure.

Some workers say that corticosteroids appear to be the most useful drugs and seem to improve the prognosis in patients particularly those with incomplete spinal cord injury. High doses are given for 2 to 4 days with gradual reduction (Kobrine *et al.* 1978, Young *et al.* 1978). Indeed, some experimental work demonstrates that animals are improved with corticosteroids (Ducker *et al.* 1969, Kuchner *et al.* 1976).

Unfortunately, the recent reports of Bracken *et al.* (1984, 1985) show that there is no proof whatsoever that corticosteroids are of any value in the treatment of acute spinal cord injury. In the first report (1984), these authors reported the absence of any effect of the high-dose of methylprednisolone sodium succinate on neurological function 6 weeks and 6 months after injury. The second report (1985) concerns a multicenter double-blind randomized clinical trial conducted by the National Acute Spinal Cord Injury Study group to examine the efficacy of high-dose methylprednisolone (1,000 mg bolus and 1,000 mg daily thereafter for 10 days) compared with that of a standard dose (100 mg bolus and 100 mg daily for 10 days). No significant difference was observed in neurological recovery 1 year after injury between the two treatment groups. Nevertheless, these results can be considered (Collins 1984).

Lesoin *et al.* (1981) use local vascular stimulants such as Piribedil (Trivastal) and Nicergoline (Sermion) in an intravenous drip, with 500 ml of isotonic glucose. The usual dose is 0.02 mg per kilogram of body weight per a day of piribedil and 0.3 mg/kg/day of nicergoline.

Gamache *et al.* (1981), Jones (1978), and Yeo *et al.* (1978) have treated acute spinal traumatic lesions within 12 hours of injuries with hyperbaric oxygenation at a pressure of 2.5 ATA. The rationale of hyperoxygenation of damaged neural tissues is the reoxygenation of those cells which are rendered hypoxic by vascular insufficiency from capillary or large vessel damage and edema. No deterioration of motor power or sensation is recorded during or after hyperbaric oxygen treatment. But, there is no evidence at all that it is beneficial.

Matinian *et al.* (1973) and Oganesian *et al.* (1964, 1971) have published reports concerning enzyme treatments in humans. In one clinical study, the enzyme preparation: Lidase (hyaluronidase) was used. Treatment begins as soon is possible, after the accident. It involves an intrathecal injection of the enzyme. Another study involved the use of a combination of two enzymes: Lidase and Trypsin. Usually, these treatments were carried out after surgery. The patients were completely paraplegic. The authors noted signs of clinical improvement long after the operation.

The enzyme therapy is considered to act by reducing the formation of scar tissue, which denies possible neuronal function. Recently, Guth *et al.* (1980) have been unable to obtain support for the contention that enzyme therapy facilitates spinal regeneration and functional recovery in spinal cord transected rats.

In conclusion, it seems that the present results in the medical treatment of acute spinal cord injuries remains poor. Indeed, no clinical study has shown a benefial effect from any of these treatments.

This should signify that what is being done does not influence the spinal cord injury.

I agree with Collins (1984) when he states that a large carefully controlled series is necessary to determine if any treatment has a beneficial effect. Thus, it is very difficult to recommend any particular treatment.

#### 3.2.3. Nerve Grafts

Many animal experiments (Wrathall *et al.* 1982) and some clinical cases in man (Patil 1981) with various grafts of nerve tissues have been described.

Today, there is no proof of their value. But, may be, regeneration of the central nervous system will become an effective therapy and will represent for the future the hopes for the recovery of spinal cord function following spinal cord injury.

### *3.3. Prevention of Complications*

Possible complications other than spinal neural, must be considered along with discussion of the treatment of osteoarticular lesions and neurological lesions. The possibility of complications and their prophylaxis must always be appreciated.

(a) Respiratory problems: These may occur, especially, if there is associated thoracic trauma.

Ventilation may be depressed by infection or atelectasis. Clinical, bacteriological, and radiological monitoring, are necessary with antibiotic therapy and possible fibro optic aspiration.

(b) Thrombo-embolic complications: Prevention involves the mobilization of the lower limbs, the use of elastic stockings, and anticoagulants usually with calciparine, and should be instituted very early in spite of the theoretical risk of haemorrhage aggravating the neural injury.

(c) Digestive complications: Paralytic ileus is not rare, and is diagnosed by abdominal meteorism. It may be treated with prostigmine associated with gastric aspiration and a rectal catheter. Later, soft laxatives are useful.

(d) Metabolic disorders: Proteinic hypercatabolism, nitrogenous escape, and anemia, can be practical problems and a daily observation of these is essential.

(e) Vegetative disorders: These are characterized by thermal and blood pressure abnormalities. They may necessitate cooling of the limbs and analgesic or anesthetic drugs.

(f) Urological problems: Urinary retention requires catheterization with strict asepsis.

It seems that the best way to treat the neuropathic bladder, certainly in the acute stage, is by intermittent catheterization. When an indwelling urethral catheter is used, both penis and catheter will be turned up over the abdomen and fixed in place in order to prevent urethritis, a periurethral abscess and a fistula.

If urinary catheterization is impossible, a catheter inserted by a suprapubic cystotomy may be required (Peatfield *et al.* 1983).

(g) Cutaneous risks: The protection of skin and the prevention of bed sores must be emphasized. The prognosis is greatly influenced by the development of pressure ulcers. They are nowadays very rare with expert nursing, and the use of appropriate beds in specialized spinal unit. We advocate particularly the BARD flotation system because of its effectiveness and low cost. We do not use the Stoke-Egerton bed or the Stryker-Frame bed in our Unit.

(h) Osteo-articular and muscular problems: Physiotherapy begins as soon as possible to prevent recumbency pathology. Daily passive mobilization of all joints is essential.

## 4. Discussion on Indications

### *4.1. Timing of Operative Treatment*

Spinal surgery includes two aspects. Either "early surgery" to realign the spinal column and to remove any compressing agents, or "late surgery" for the clear indication of achieving spinal stability with internal fixation by devices and/or fusion with bone.

Many neurosurgeons prefer emergency surgery; others, "as soon as possible".

Indeed, the Allen's (1917) experimental studies suggest that the majority of the destructive process, in the injured spinal cord, appear to occur within 4–8 hours following trauma, and most of the experimental therapy to decrease the resulting deficit is only effective if it is applied within these first few hours.

Others experimental studies have supported this hypothesis and have been a major impetus for early surgical treatment. Thus, Bedoiseau *et al.* (1971) state that thoracic and lumbar spine injuries necessitate emergency surgery for spinal reduction and stabilization, more so than for cervical spine injuries. They insist on surgery before six hours following injury. What is important is emergency reduction of fractures and fracture-dislocations either by orthopedic or neurosurgical specialists.

Louis (1975) carries out on emergency orthopedic reduction followed by immobilization in a plaster corset, which allows some time for possible delayed surgical treatment if this is indicated. Brunon *et al.* (1973) agree. When there are severe neurological signs, they perform an emergency orthopedic reduction. Shock and associated injuries are treated. If reduction is not obtained by their treatment, open surgery is immediately undertaken. When neurological signs are minimal or absent, orthopedic or surgical reduction takes place as soon as possible to prevent complications. Perves *et al.* (1973) also advise emergency reduction particularly in cases of injuries of the thoraco-lumbar junction and lumbar spine with neurological signs. Reduction is followed by surgical fixation as rapidly as possible.

Jacobs *et al.* (1980), in the majority of patients, perform operative treatment as soon as the patient's condition is suitable. For us, operative treatment should be considered as an emergency, i.e., within 24 hours when spinal malignment cannot be corrected, a partial neurological injury involves the cord, or the deficit progresses. In patients who have little or no neurologic deficit and whose spinal malignment has been reduced by postural means, stabilization can be deferred (in their series, it was deferred for an average of 5 days).

Several authors recommend early "aggressive" treatment (Burke *et al.* 1976, Lagarrigues *et al.* 1980, Lesoin *et al.* 1980), especially for lesions at the thoraco-lumbar junction, where a combination of spinal cord and cauda equina injury is present (Erickson *et al.* 1977).

But it is a fact that no treatment can be demonstrated to be more effective than any other treatment (Collins 1984).

Thus, Dickson *et al.* (1978) in most of these patients perform Harrington instrumentation and fusion, and they compare patients who had the operation on the day of injury and those who did not have it until eight to thirty-five days later, to see if there was a difference between the degree of neural recovery in two groups. The two groups were compared with regards to age, cause of injury, fracture level, angle of deformity and displacement. The groups appeared to be approximately comparable. The conclusion was that the return of neural function was the same in each group. Nevertheless, although some patients with severe injuries should not undergo immediate surgery, they advocate reduction and stabilization as an emergency procedure on the day of injury if at all possible.

In the same way, Flesch *et al.* (1977) analyze their cases to determine if there is any correlation between the extent of neural recovery and the timing of decompression. They discover that there is no difference in the extent of neural recovery in patients with incomplete or cauda equina lesions treated by immediate, early, or late decompression and that complete lesions remain unchanged whatever the timing of the decompression.

These data, and the fact that an emergency treatment which causes a second injury may do harm, support the concept of a delayed surgical procedure after a varied period of conservative treatment, usually from 7–15 days (Jelsma *et al.* 1982, Schmidek *et al.* 1980, Larson *et al.* 1976). Also, in these patients associated injuries are often a major contraindication to immediate or early spinal surgical intervention.

Personally, I agree with this attitude. But early operative treatment is necessary for certain fractures of the lumbar spine with neurological deficit, in which myelography reveals dural and arachnoid tears and prolapse of cauda equina roots (Harris 1977, Miller 1980).

The evidence of improved neurological function with decompressive procedures and/or fracture reduction and stabilization, either immediate or delayed, is not at all conclusive.

### *4.2. Different Methods of Treatment*

The indications for the different methods appear to be related to two kinds of problems:

(a) Orthopedic problems, depending on the type and the level of the lesion, and the stability.

(b) Neurological problems, related to the presence of neurological signs, or with the risk of delayed neural injury.

In a simplified manner, from the bony point of view, stable fractures will be managed by orthopedic means, and unstable lesions will be operated upon. However, there is a problem to clearly define the notion of stability or instability, varying between different authors, and the different anatomical and functional interpretations. Some advocate orthopedic treatment alone and others prefer a systematic surgical attitude in most patients.

Concerning these attitudes, certain aspects may be emphasized:

1) Fracture-dislocations and burst fractures are usually considered to be unstable, and will be amenable to open surgery; and the presence of a retropulsed bone or/and disc fragment into the spinal canal as demonstrated by a CT scan is an additional argument for surgery.

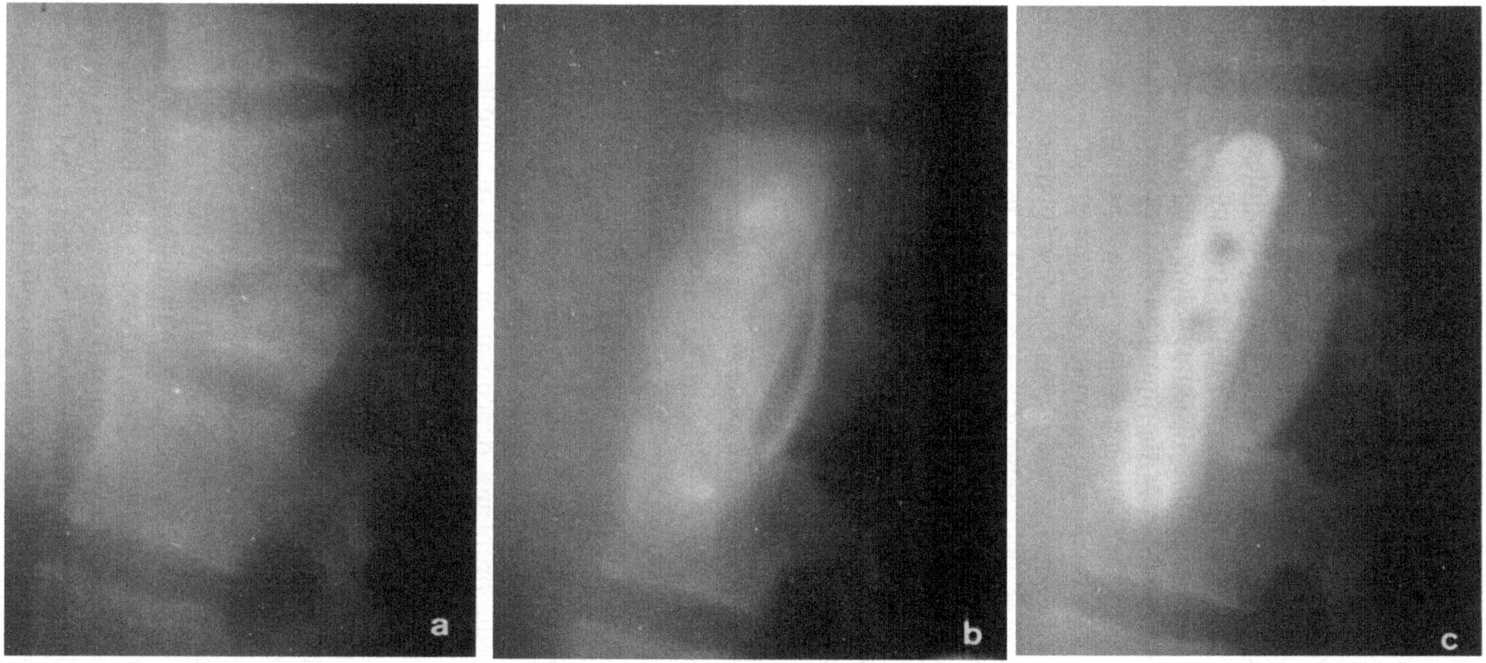


Fig. 8. Severe burst fracture of L 1 without neurological signs operated one month after a traffic accident. Antero-lateral approach; intercorporeal iliac bone graft. Instrumentation with Roy-Camille plates

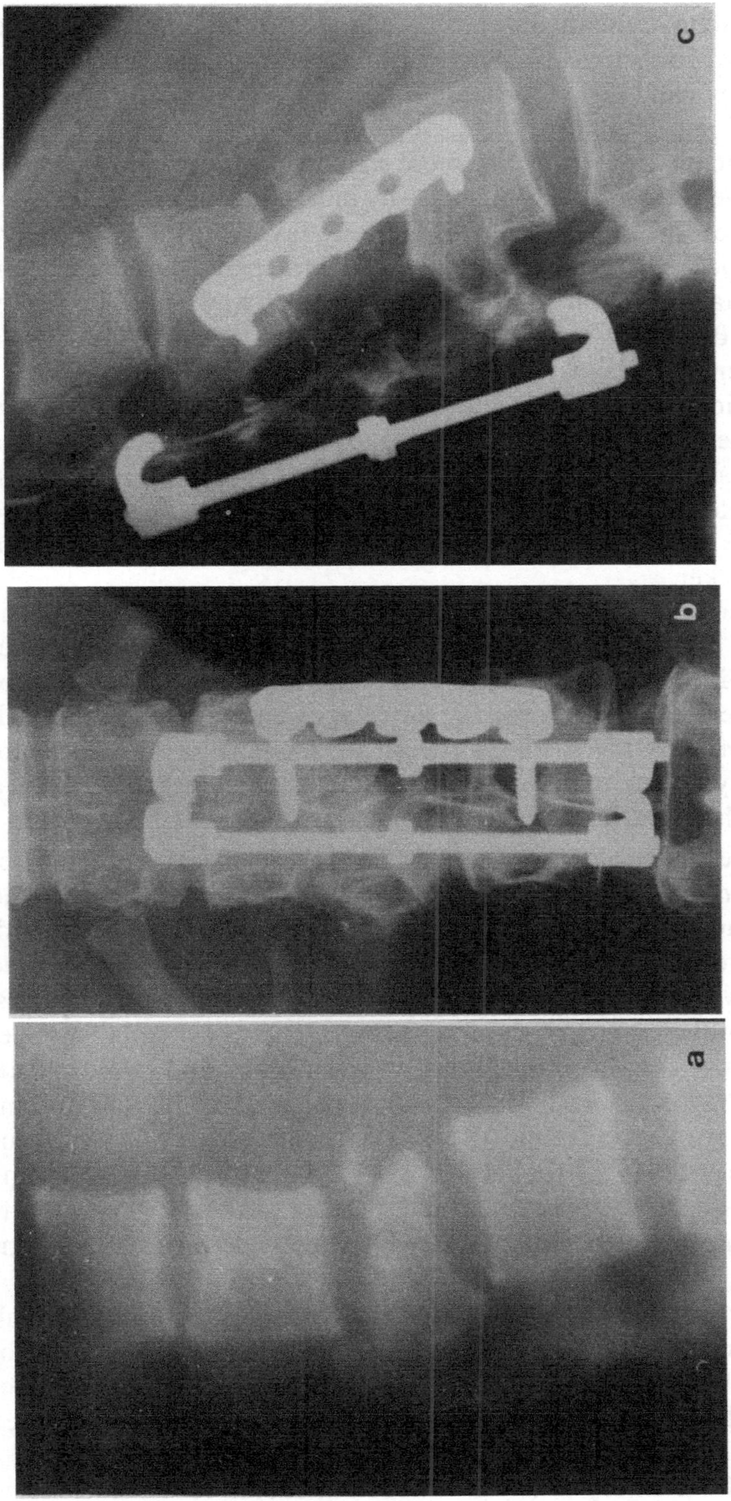


Fig. 9. Severe burst fracture of L 2. Incomplete cauda equina syndrome. Mixed approach. First a posterior approach and fixation with Knodt compression instrumentation, then an antero-lateral approach 15 days later; corporectomy, iliac bone graft and Roy-Camille plates screwed into the L 1 and L 3 vertebrae. Complete neurological recovery

2) Wedge-fractures are usually considered to be stable and will be treated by conservative, non-surgical means with changes in accordance to the degree of kyphosis and the importance of anterior bony wedge; in patients without neurological abnormalities, the minor wedge lesions by immobilization and physiotherapy; the more significant wedge lesions involving a third of the vertebral body or more, by immobilization with a plaster corset in hyperlordosis; the major wedge lesions, involving more than 50% of the antero-posterior diameter of the vertebral body, and which are potentially unstable, by Harrington instrumentation and spinal fusion by some workers (Bradford *et al.* 1977); by others by external reduction if the posterior elements and spinal canal are not injured (Seljeskog 1982).

3) The flexion-distraction fractures (Chance's fractures) are usually considered to be stable, without any risk to nervous structures, and will be treated by a plaster in lordosis (O'Callaghan *et al.* 1980, Rennie *et al.* 1973). However, Fuentes *et al.* (1984) advocate open surgery for the lesions of type I, II, III, and for the lesions of type IV, an external fixation in lordosis with a plaster body jacket.

When the choice is surgical, the kind of approach, the type of arthrodesis with or without an associated bony fusion, depends essentially on personal bias. Patients with an isolated corporeal and discal lesion without injury of the posterior elements, do best with an anterior or antero-lateral approach (Chabannes *et al.* 1982) (Fig. 8); and lesions of the posterior elements are best managed by a posterior approach. In complex lesions of the vertebra, a mixed approach, is considered (Figs. 9 and 10).

The presence of neurological signs influences the choice of the method of treatment according to two factors: the severity of neurological signs and the level of injury. When patients have complete lesions of the spinal cord, there is no prospect of useful neurological recovery, whether treated surgically by whatever means or managed conservatively. Nevertheless, surgery can provide secure stabilization and may promote speedier rehabilitation and avoid complications of recumbency and late displacements (Hardy 1965, Norrell 1978). With partial spinal cord lesions conservative treatment may lead to some neurological recovery in some patients (Burke *et al.* 1975, Frankel *et al.* 1969, Guttmann 1973). According to some authors, early decompression and stabilization of the spine appears to encourage maximal neurological recovery (Brunon *et al.* 1973, Kobrine *et al.* 1978).

It is said that the proportion of patients who had virtually full neurological recovery is greater in the series of surgically treated cases of Larson *et al.* (1976) than in the series of conservatively managed cases of Frankel *et al.* (1969); however, the data must be examined and considered with very great care.

The level of the injury is a very important factor to consider when neurological signs are present. Thus, lesions of the thoraco-lumbar junction and lesions of the lumbar spine necessitate emergency reduction with early stabilization, on the other hand injuries with complete neurological loss are an indication for non-surgical treatment according to some authors (Perves

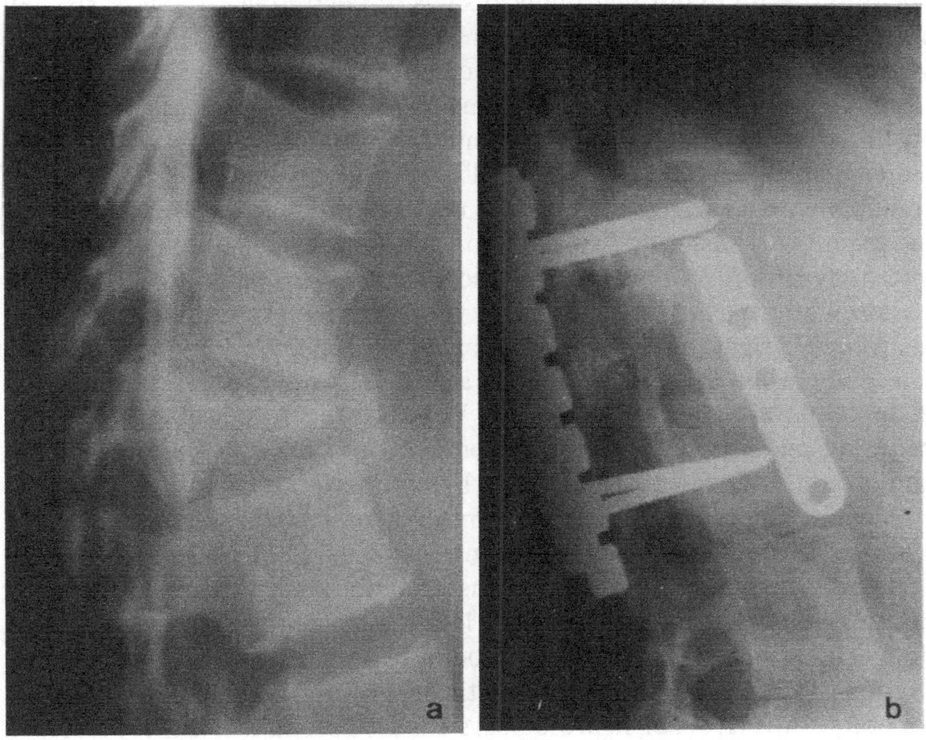

Fig. 10. Severe burst fracture of T 12. Complete paraplegia. Mixed approach. First a posterior approach. Short immobilization with Roy-Camille's plates, then an antero-lateral approach. Corporectomy, iliac bone graft, and instrumentation with Roy-Camille plates

*et al.* 1973) because the lesions are relatively stable and the likelihood of recovery is minimal.

When both the anatomical aspects of the bony lesion and neurological signs are considered, some recommendations may be discussed. Thus Louis *et al.* (1975) prefer posterior surgical fixation for unstable fractures of paraplegic patients if there is no narrowing of the spinal canal and no corporeal defect after orthopedic reduction. Anterior decompression is reserved for lesions with a narrowed spinal canal and/or a bony defect after reduction, and the mixed approach both posterior and anterior is reserved for very unstable fractures with an anterior bony defect and with narrowing of the spinal canal.

Terver (1975) proposes the following plan:

In patients with anterior "vertical" instability by a corporo-discal lesion with important neurological signs, an emergency posterior approach with laminectomy and instrumentation, and posterior interbody fusion are performed at the same time, or an antero-lateral procedure at a subsequent operation. With minor neurological signs or delayed neurological risk; an antero-lateral approach for decompression and bone graft is recommend. Without neurological signs: the orthopedic technique of Böhler (1944). If there is a lesion of the horizontal elements on which ligaments and muscles are inserted, open surgery by an anterior approach and bony fusion is recommended. In case of "horizontal" instability by lesions of the articular columns with neurological signs or neurological risk: the recommended procedure is a posterior approach for laminectomy, instrumentation and interbody fusion. Without neurological signs: instrumentation alone by a posterior approach. Mixed instability with complex lesions of vertebrae and neurological signs: a posterior approach for laminectomy, instrumentation interbody fusion at the same time, or a secondary anterior interbody fusion if the corporeal injury is dominant. Withouth neurological signs or with neurological risk: a posterior approach for instrumentation without laminectomy. Then subsequent interbody antero-lateral fusion.

When complex lesions are responsible for mixed instability and are associated with paraplegia, Chabannes *et al.* (1982) prefer a posterior approach for laminectomy and instrumentation; a bone graft being debateable. When the neurological lesion is incomplete, they propose a double approach separated by a period of two weeks. The first procedure is a laminectomy and instrumentation, the second an antero-lateral operation for bony grafting. When neurological signs are absent, they either perform a double approach, or only an antero-lateral approach with a longer period of immobilization.

## 5. Results

### *5.1. Neurological Results*

Many authors state that there is no significant difference in eventual neurological recovery whether patients are treated by conservative measures or by surgery. Flesch *et al.* (1977) observed that complete lesions remained unchanged whatever the timing of decompression, and that the type of initial decompression and its extent did no appear to influence neural recovery. Bedoiseau *et al.* (1971) and Lagarrigues *et al.* (1980) state that incomplete neurological signs "are not made worse by surgery".

### *5.2. Orthopedic Results*

The orthopedic result depends both on stability and on the quality of reduction. Early mobilization is essential.

According to Jacobs *et al.* (1980), anatomical results are assessed by antero-posterior and lateral X-rays. Less than 10% displacement and 15° for angulation is considered to be an anatomical reduction.

Lesoin *et al.* (1982) judge the results good if the kyphosis is less than or equal to 15°, and the posterior wall is receded less than 2 mm.

Osebold *et al.* (1981) compare six different treatment groups and conclude that the greatest increase in angulation compared to preoperative values is seen in patients treated without an operation. The groups showing a decrease in angulation and the greatest improvement in anterior displacement is obtained in those treated surgically, particularly by fusion and fixation instrumentation. Optimal stability as shown by flexion-extension X-ray views is seen in patients operated on. It should be remembered that Nicoll (1949) found that anatomical reduction is not necessary for a good functional result. He reported on 166 patients who had been working for at least two years following injury, and who had sustained severe spinal deformities. But in his series, there was a high proportion of patients with back pain in nonoperated patients.

I personally prefer to restore correct anatomical continuity of the spinal column either with positioning, or by a delayed external or surgical technique.

### *5.3. Complications*

(a) General: Several important complications are related to recumbency, such as thrombo-embolic and urinary and respiratory, and require expert preventative and therapeutic measures. In the series of Jacobs *et al.* (1980), the complication rate was 18% in 32 recumbently treated patients and in contrast, in 55 patients treated with Harrington instrumentation, the complication rate was 7%.

(b) Related to the type of treatment: Some complications are common to both orthopedic and surgical treatment (pain and stiffness in the patient's back, progressive angular kyphosis, pseudarthrosis), others are specific to surgery (infection, particularly when metallic instrumentation is applied to the spine) and depend also on the instrumentation used (screws broken with Roy-Camille's plates, rods broken and hooks displaced with Harrington). Because of the frequency and character pain necessitates particular consideration. The problem concerns both pain in relation to the spinal injury and which requires various therapies (analgesics, transcutaneous stimulator) (Nepomuceno *et al.* 1979), and pain as a complication related to the surgical treatment of spinal cord injury patients. Mild back pain is typically described at the site of surgery.

Osebold *et al.* (1981) state that pain is commoner in patients who have had a laminectomy than for those without such treatment. Moreover, the incidence of pain in laminectomized patients increase with the number of levels operated.

Burke (1973) notes a probable relationship between chronic spinal pain in paraplegics and posterior spinal surgery, particularly laminectomy. In a group of 115 patients, Burke (1976) reported that ten complained of chronic severe spinal pain; out of eighty-nine patients treated conservatively, only two (2%) had chronic pain, compared to eight of twenty-six surgically treated patients (22%). All eight surgically treated patients with pain had had posterior operations. Similarly, Roberts (1970) points out that pain occurs in 40% of patients with unstable fractures treated by laminectomy, without reduction and fusion.

Osebold *et al.* (1981), Lewis and Mc Kibbin (1974) and Nicoll (1949) found a high incidence of pain in their nonoperated patients. Nicoll (1949) reported that of his nonoperative patients with fracture dislocations, 43% had pain at the fracture site, and 57% had low-back pain. In their series of forty patients with unstable thoraco-lumbar fractures treated with Harrington instrumentation and spine fusion, Flesch *et al.* (1977) note only a 10% incidence of back pain. They state that reduction and instrumentation and fusion appear to decrease the likelihood of later back symptoms. On the other hand, among patients who had fusion and instrumentation, there is an increase in pain incidence with the number of levels instrumented.

My personal impression is that "long" versus "short" fusion and instrumentation increases the incidence of back pain. In the instrumented cases, the development of pain within 1 year usually necessitates request removal of the plates or rods.

## 6. "How to Do It"

From what I have said, it appears very difficult to generalize concerning the optimal management, however, I would like to present some ideas from a study of 168 patients with thoraco-lumbar spine fractures.

Precise and repeated clinical evaluation is necessary to classify the injured patient and appreciate the prognosis. A somatosensory evoked potential study, should be done if possible as it permits a better determination of neural lesions and also of prognosis. Emergency radiographic studies must include standard X-rays views, and lateral and antero-posterior tomographic sections. These demonstrate the features of the lesion, the stability, and the presence of retropulsed bone and/or disc fragments into the spinal canal. Data from CT scans are essential to determine the dimensions of the spinal canal and to visualize precisely an intracanalar bony fragment. Metrizamide myelography is useful to provide an explanation for a neurological deficit if the vertebral lesions are inadequate to explain such a deficit. In such patients, an epidural haematoma or a herniated disc must be suspected.

Our indication are varied, if we consider the following distribution (Table 1):

Table 1. *Treatment of 168 Thoraco-Lumbar Spine Fractures*

| | |
|---|---|
| External techniques | 25% |
| Open surgery | 52% |
| Conservative management | 23% |

44 patients were treated by external techniques, and 90 underwent open surgery; 34 were managed conservatively because of their serious condition partly because of multiple injuries, partly in relation to the severity of their neurological state. We operate on lesions considered to be unstable, i.e., fracture-dislocation, burst fractures and wedge fractures involving more than 50% of the anterior-posterior body diameter. The unstable character of a burst or wedge fracture is nowadays better estimated, when the CT scan demonstrates disruption of both the anterior and the posterior segments of the vertebra. The aim of surgical intervention is to achieve stabilization. In our series (Table 2) a classical posterior approach is used in 70% of operated patients with installation of Roy-Camille's plates in the majority of cases (60%). Nowadays, the surgical procedure is delayed after a period of conservative treatment, usually 7–15 days if a neurological deficit is present, less without such an abnormality.

Table 2. *Surgical Treatment of 88 Thoraco-Lumbar Spine Lesions*

| | |
|---|---|
| Classic posterior approach | 70% |
| With Roy-Camille's plates | 60% |
| Anterior approach | 14% |
| Combined approach | 16% |
| Laminectomy | 42% |
| Bone graft | 33% |

Previously, we have tried to proceed with surgery (within 24 hours) in all patients with neurological signs. Reduction and instrumentation was performed, at the same operations, usually with Roy-Camille's plates. We note any definite improvement in the neurological status, and also any postoperative neurological deterioration.

However, it is certain that inappropriate treatment may cause a second injury and do harm. Sometimes early surgery is required, particularly in certain patients with lumbar spine fractures with partial neurological deficit where myelography reveals dural tears and prolapse of roots.

In the recent times, we have operated on patients with severe wedge or burst fractures with intracanalar bony fragments and a significantly narrowed spinal canal diagnosed on CT scan. In these patients there is a delayed neurological risk if the vertebral angulation increases. Surgery consists initially of a posterior arthrodesis with Roy-Camille's plates, and then a delayed operation with an anterior decompression and bone graft.

In our series surgical management was used mainly for injuries of the thoraco-lumbar and the lumbar-spine, and the conservative treatment for lesions of the thoracic spine.

The kind of surgical approach depends on the nature of the vertebral lesion (Table 2).

Schematically, if corporeo-discal lesions are severe and predominant, the approach will be antero-lateral; if lesions are posterior, the approach will be posterior. When injuries are complex, two operations, with an interval of about 15 days are recommended, the posterior being first. The instrumentation varies with the biomechanical aspect of fracture. The Knodt compression instrumentation is particularly well adapted for predominant posterior lesions as in flexion distraction injuries. In the majority of other lesions, the instrumentation of Roy-Camille is very effective.

Bone graft fusion is used when the approach is anterior, after the removal of a disc or after corporectomy. For posterior instrumentation, fusion is considered.

After surgery, a plaster corset allows early mobilization, within ten days. The corset is retained for twelve weeks. This type of management usually promotes speedier rehabilitation, easier nursing care and decreased recumbency complications.

## References

1. Allen AR (1914) Remarks on the histopathological changes in the spinal cord due to impact. An experimental study. J Nerv Ment Dis 41: 141 – 147
2. Beattie FC (1969) Distraction rod fusion. Clin Orthop 62: 218 – 222
3. Bedbrook GM (1969) Use and disuse of surgery in lumbo-dorsal fractures. J Western Pacific Orthop Assoc 6: 5 – 26
4. Bedoiseau M, Roy-Camille R, Roy-Camille M, Saillant G (1971) Examen clinique d'un traumatisé récent de la moelle. Conclusions pronostiques et thérapeutiques immédiates. Rev Prat 21 (25): 3707 – 3728
5. Benassy J, Blanchard J, Lecog P (1967) Neurological recovery rate in para- and tetraplegia. Paraplegia 4: 259 – 269
6. Boehler J (1944) Technique du traitement des fractures. Masson, Paris, pp 255 – 382
7. Boehler J (1956) The treatment of fractures, ed 5, vol 1. Grune and Stratton, New York

8. Boehler J (1970) Operative treatment of fractures of the dorsal and lumbar spine. J Trauma 10: 1119–1122
9. Bohlman HH (1974) Traumatic fractures of the upper thoracic spinal with paraplegia. J Bone Joint Surg 56 A: 1299
10. Bracken MB, Collins WF, Freeman DF *et al* (1984) Efficacy of methylprednisolone in acute spinal cord injury. JAMA 251: 45–52
11. Bracken MB, Shepard MJ, Hellenbrand KG *et al* (1985) Methylprednisolone and neurological function 1 year after spinal cord injury. Results of the national acute spinal cord injury study. Volume 63: No 5, 704–713
12. Bradford DS, Behrooz A, Winter RB, Seljeskog EL (1977) Surgical stabilization of fracture and fracture-dislocations of the thoracic spine. Spine 2: 185–196
13. Bradford DS, Thompson RC (1976) Fractures and dislocations of the spine: Indications for surgical interventions. Minn Med 58: 711–720
14. Brant-Zawadzki M, Brooke R Jr, Hideyo M, Pitts LH (1982) High resolution CT of thoraco lumbar fractures. AJR 138: 699–704
15. Brant-Zawadzki M, Miller EM, Federle MP (1981) CT in the evaluation of spine trauma. AJR 136: 369–375
16. Bricolo A, Dalle Ore G, Da Pian R, Faccioli F (1976) Local cooling in spinal cord injury. Surg Neurol 6 (2): 101–106
17. Brunon J, Goutelle A, Felman D, Bret P, Ravon R (1973) Résultats et indications de l'ostéosynthèse postérieure par plaques métalliques dans les fractures du rachis. Neurochirurgie 19 (2): 199–213
18. Burke DC (1973) Pain in paraplegia. Paraplegia 10: 297–313
19. Burke DC, Murray DD (1975) The management of thoracic and thoracolumbar injuries of the spine with neurological involvement. J Bone Joint Surg 57: 254
20. Burke DC, Duncan M (1976) The management of thoracic and thoracolumbar injuries of the spine with neurological involvement. J Bone Joint Surg 58 (1): 72–78
21. Bussat P, Rossier AB, Djindjian R, Vasey H, Berney J (1973) Spinal cord angiography in dorsolumbar vertebral fractures with neurological involvement. Radiology 109: 617–620
22. Carey PC (1965) Neurosurgery and paraplegia. Rehabilitation 52: 27–29
23. Carson J, Gumpert J, Jefferson A (1971) Diagnosis and treatment of thoracic intervertebral disc protrusions. J Neurol Neurosurg Psychiatry 34: 68–77
24. Chabannes J, Floucaud D, Colnet G, Paquet F (1982) Notre expérience des greffes vertébrales dans la chirurgie des fractures graves récentes du rachis dorso-lobaire. Neurochirurgie 28: 235–244
25. Chance GQ (1948) Note on a type of flexion fracture of the spine. Br J Radiol 21: 452–453
26. Chehrazi B, Wagner FC, Collins WF, Freeman DH (1981) A scale for evaluation of spinal cord injuries. J Neurosurg 54: 310–315
27. Chengqi W (1979) Antero-lateral decompression for spinal fractures complicated by paraplegia. Clin Med J 92: 149–154
28. Chou SN (1978) Treatment of thoracic spinal deformities with neurologic

deficit. In: Chou SN, Seljeskog, EL (eds) Spinal deformity in neurological dysfunction. Raven Press, New York, pp 131–137
29. Cloward RB (1963) Lesions of the intervertebral discs and their treatment by interbody fusion methods. Clin Orthop 27: 57–77
30. Colley DP, Dunsker SB (1978) Traumatic narrowing of the dorso-lumbar spinal canal demonstrated by computed tomography. Radiology 129: 95–98
31. Collins WF (1983) A review and update of experiment and clinical studies of spinal cord injury. Paraplegia 21: 204–219
32. Collins WF (1984) A review of treatment of spinal cord injury. Br J Surg 71 (12): 974–975
33. Convery FR, Minteer MA, Smith RW, Emerson SM (1978) Fracture-dislocation of the dorsal lumbar spine. Acute operative stabilization by Harrington instrumentation. Spine 3 (2): 160–166
34. Creyssel J (1950) Ostéosynthèse vertébrale suivant la technique de Wilson. Mém de l'acad Chir 76 (1, 2, 3): 160–166
35. Cusick JF, Myklebust JB, Larson SH, Sances A Jr (1979) Spinal cord evaluation by cortical evoked responses. Arch Neurol 36: 140–143
36. Davis AG (1938) Tensile strength of the anterior longitudinal ligament in relation to treatment of 132 crush fractures of the spine. J Bone Joint Surg 20: 429–438
37. Decoulx P, Rieunau G (1958) Les fractures du rachis dorso-lombaire sans troubles nerveux. Rev Chir Orthop 44 (3–4): 254–322
38. Decoulx P, Soulier A, Waghemacker R (1955) Paraplégie traumatique. Laminectomie et Wilson. Lille Chir 10: 245–252
39. Decoulx P, Rieunau G (1959) Les fractures du rachis dorso-lombaire sans troubles nerveux. Rev Chir Orthop 45 (2): 237–294
40. Dickson JH, Harrington PR, Erwin WD (1973) Harrington instrumentation in the fractured unstable thoracic and lumbar spine. Tex Med 69: 91–98
41. Dickson H, Harrington PR, Wendell DE (1978) Results of reduction and stabilization of the severely fractured thoracic and lumbar spine. J Bone Joint Surg 60 (6): 799–805
42. Dohn F (1979) Thoracic spinal cord decompression: Alternative surgical approaches and basis of choise. Clin Neurosurg 27: 611–623
43. Doppman JL, Girton M (1976) Angiographic study of the effect of laminectomy in the presence of acute anterior epidural masses. J Neurosurg 45: 195–202
44. Ducker TB, Hamit HF (1969) Experimental treatments of acute spinal cord injury. J Neurosurg 30: 693–697
45. Durward QJ, Schweigel JF, Harrison P (1981) Management of fractures of the thoracolumbar and lumbar spine. Neurosurgery 8 (5): 555–561
46. Dwyer AF, Newton NC, Sherwood AA (1969) An anterior approach to scoliosis. Clin Orthop 62: 192–202
47. Erickson DL (1978) Treatment of thoracolumbar fractures with associated neurological injury. In: Chou SN, Seljeskog EL (eds) Spinal deformities and neurological dysfunction. Raven Press, New York, pp 139–146
48. Erickson L, Leider LL Jr, Brown WE (1977) One stage decompression-stabilization for thoraco-lumbar fractures. Spine 2 (1): 53–56

49. Flamm ES, Young W, Demepoulos HB *et al* (1982) Experimental spinal cord injury: treatment with naloxone. J Neurosurg 10: 227 – 231
50. Flesch JR, Leider LL, Erickson DL, Chou SN, Bradford DS (1977) Harrington instrumentation and spine fusion for thoracic and lumbar spine fractures. J Bone Joint Surg 59 (2): 143 – 153
51. Fountain SS, Nagel DA, Jameson RM (1978) Complications from Harrington distraction rod fixation of fracture dislocation of the spine. Proceedings of société internationale de chirurgie orthopédique et de traumatologie. Kyoto, Japon, p 182
52. Frankel HL, Hancock DO, Hyslop G, Melzak J, Michaelis LS, Ungar GH, Vernon JDS, Walsh JJ (1969) The value of postural reduction in the initial management of closed injuries of the spine with paraplegia and tetraplegia. Paraplegia 7: 179 – 192
53. Fuentes JM, Bonnel F (1984) Le vissage pédiculaire du rachis lombaire bas (L 3 – L 4 – L 5) et de la charnière lombo-sacrée. Rev Chir Orthop 70: 479 – 482
54. Fuentes JM, Bloncourt J, Bourbotte G, Castan Ph, Vlahovitch B (1984) La fracture de Chance. Neurochirurgie 30: 113 – 118
55. Gage EL, Shim NK, Ransohoff J (1969) Anterior approach to acute and chronic thoraco-lumbar spinal cord compression. Proceedings of the 17th veterans administration spinal cord injury conference, Bronx, NY, pp 45 – 50
56. Gamache FW, Myers Ram, Ducker TB, Cowley RA (1981) The clinical application of hyperbaric oxygen therapy in spinal cord injury: A preliminary report. Surg Neurol 15 (2): 85 – 87
57. Geisler WO, Wynne-Jones J, Jousee AT (1966) Early management of the patient with trauma to the spinal cord. Med Serv J Can 22: 512 – 523
58. Gonon G, Rousson B, Fischer L, Mourgues G (1974) Intérêt chirurgical de la connaissance anatomique des directions pédiculaires au niveau du rachis dorso-lombaire. Lyon Chir 70: 408 – 410
59. Grantham SA, Malberg M, Smith DM (1976) Thoraco-lumbar spine flexion-distraction injure. Spine 1: 172 – 177
60. Guth L, Albuquerque EX, Deshpande SS, Barrett CP, Donati EJ, Warnick J (1980) Ineffectiveness of enzyme therapy on regeneration in the transected spinal cord of the rat. J Neurosurg 52: 73 – 86
61. Guttmann L (1949) Surgical aspects of the treatment of traumatic paraplegia. J Bone Joint Surg 31 B: 399 – 403
62. Guttmann L (1954) Initial treatment of traumatic paraplegia. Proc R Soc Med 47: 1103 – 1109
63. Guttmann L (1969) Spinal deformities in traumatic paraplegics and tetraplegics following surgical procedures. Paraplegia 7: 38 – 58
64. Guttmann L (1973) Spinal cord injuries; comprehensive management and research. Blackwell, Oxford, pp 151 – 176
65. Hardy AG (1965) The treatment of paraplegia due to fracture-dislocations of the dorso-lumbar spine. Paraplegia 3: 112 – 123
66. Harrington PR (1967) Instrumentation in spine instability other than scoliosis. S Afr J Surg 5: 7 – 12

67. Harrington PR, Dickson JH (1973) The development and further prospects of internal fixation of the spine. Isr J Med Sci 9: 773–778
68. Harris P (1963) Proceedings of the symposium on spinal injuries Royal College of Surgeons, Edinburgh, Scotland, p 105
69. Harris Ph (1977) Closed injuries of the dorsal and dorso-lumbar spine and cord. Proceedings of an international medical faculty. "On the acute management of spinal injuries". Sir Guttmann L (ed). Published by the veterans Administration, Washington DC, USA, pp 150–152
70. Herrmann HD (1979) Transarticular (transpedicular) metal plate fixation for stabilization of the lumbar and thoracic spine. Acta Neurochir (Wien) 48: 101–110
71. Hodgson AR, Stock FE (1956) Anterior spinal fusion: Preliminary communication on the radical treatment of Pott's disease and Pott's paraplegia. Br J Surg 2: 266–275
72. Holdsworth FW (1963) Early orthopedic treatment of patients with spinal injury. Proceedings of a symposium held in the royal college of surgeons of Edinburgh. Morrison and Gibb, Edinburgh, Scotland, pp 93–101
73. Holdsworth (1963) Fractures-dislocations of the spine. J Bone Joint Surg 45 B (1): 6–20
74. Holdsworth F (1970) Fractures, dislocations and fractures-dislocations of the spine. J Bone Joint Surg 52 A (8): 1534–1552
75. Holdsworth FW, Hardy A (1953) Early treatment of paraplegia from fractures of the thoracic-lumbar spine. J Bone Joint Surg 35 B: 540–550
76. Houdart R, Guillaumat M, Maury M (1973) La chirurgie d'urgence dans les traumatismes vertébromédullaires fermés. Nouv Presse Méd 2 (35): 2331–2334
77. Jacobs R, Asher MA, Snider RK (1980) Thoraco-lumbar spinal injuries A comparative study of recumbent and operative treatment in 100 patients. Spine 5 (5): 463–477
78. Jelsma RK, Kirsch PT, Jelsma LF, Ramsey WC, Rice JF (1982) Surgical treatment of thoraco-lumbar fractures. Surg Neurol 18 (3): 156–166
79. Jones FR (1978) Hyperbaric oxygen and acute spinal cord injuries in humans. Med J Aust 2 (12): 573–575
80. Katznelson AA (1969) Stabilization of the spine in traumatic paraplegia. Paraplegia 6: 33–37
81. Kaufer H, Hayes JT (1966) Lumbar fracture-dislocation. A study of twenty-one cases. J Bone Joint Surg 48 A: 712–730
82. Kelly RP, Whitesides TE Jr (1968) Treatment of lumbo-dorsal fracture-dislocations. Ann Surg 167: 705–717
83. Kempf I, Briot B, Fernandez M, Grosse A, Renard M (1973) Le traitement des traumatismes vertébro-médullaires. Intérêt de la fixation des fractures et fractures-luxations du rachis dorso-lombaire à l'aide du matériel de Harrington "en compression". Rev Chir Orthop 59: 477–489
84. Kempf I, Jaeger JH, Briot B, Lemaguet A (1977) L'ostéosynthèse en compression des fractures et fractures-luxations du rachis par le matériel de Harrington inversé. Rev Chir Orthop 63: 458–462

85. Kobrine AI, Stopak B (1978) Advances in the treatment of thoracolumbar injuries. Clin Neurosurg 26: 570–581
86. Kuchner EF, Hansebout RR (1976) Combined steroid and hypothermia treatment of experimental spinal cordinjury. Surg Neurol 6: 371–376
87. Lafferty JF, Winter WG, Gambaro SA (1977) Fatigue characteristics of posterior elements of vertebrae. J Bone Joint Surg 59: 154–158
88. Lagarrigues *et al.* (1980) Plaques vissées et fractures du rachis dorso-lombaire. Rev Med (Toulouse) 16: 99–107
89. Larson SJ (1979) Unstable thoracic fractures: Treatment alternatives and the role of the neurosurgeons. Clin Neurosurg 27: 624–640
90. Larson SJ, Holst RA, Hemmy DC, Sances A Jr (1976) Lateral extracavitary approach to traumatic lesions of the thoracic and lumbar spine. J Neurosurg 45: 628–637
91. Larson SJ, Sances A Jr, Christenson PC (1966) Evoked somatosensory potentials in man. Arch Neurol 15: 88–93
92. Lesoin F, Bouasakao N, Cama A, Lozes G, Combelles G (1982) Post-traumatic fixation of the thoraco lumbar spine using Roy-Camille plates. Surg Neurol 18 (3): 167–173
93. Lesoin F, Bouasakao N, Jomin N (1984) Voie d'abord antéro-interne du rachis lombaire. Neurochirurgie 30: 433–436
94. Lewis J, Mc Kibbin B (1974) The treatment of unstable fracture-dislocations of the thoraco-lumbar spine accompanied by paraplegia. J Bone Joint Surg 56 B: 603–612
95. Louis R (1974) Voie d'abord de la charnière dorso-lombaire. Les conférences d'enseignement. SOFCOT Paris 1973. L'expansion scientique, Paris, pp 96–127
96. Louis R (1977) Symposium sur les fractures instables du rachis. Les théories de l'instabilité. 51e réunion annuelle de la SOFCOT, 1976. Rev Chir Orthop 63: 423–425
97. Louis R (1982) Chirurgie du rachis. Anatomie chirurgicale et voies d'abord. Springer, Berlin Heidelberg New York
98. Louis R, Bonsignour JP, Ouiminga R (1975) Les fractures du rachis: une attitude thérapeutique à propos d'une série de 100 cas. Méditerranée 80: 81–106
99. Mallet-Guy P (1938) Le traitement non sanglant des fractures du rachis, fractures récentes, fractures anciennes, techniques et résultats. Masson, Paris
100. Menard V (1984) Causas de la paraplégie dans le mal de Pott. Rev Orthop 5: 47–64
101. Michel CR, Onimus M (1977) L'utilisation du matériel de Harrington en détraction dans le traitement des fractures du rachis. Symposium sur les fractures instables du rachis. 51e réunion annuelle de la SOFCOT, 1976. Rev Chir Orthop 63: 456–458
102. Miller CA, Dewey RC, Hunt WE (1980) Impaction fracture of the lumbar vertebral with dural tear. J Neurosurg 53: 765–771
103. Morgan Th, Wharton GW, Austin GN (1971) The results of laminectomy in patients with incomplete spinal cord injuries. Paraplegia 9: 14–23

104. Naidich TP, Pudlowski RM, Moran CJ, Gilula LA, Murphy W, Naidich JB (1979) Computed tomography of spinal fractures. Adv Neurol 22: 207 – 253
105. Nash CL Jr, Schatzinger LH, Brown RH, Brodkey J (1977) The unstable stable thoracic compression fracture. Spine 2: 261 – 265
106. Matinian LA, Andreasian AS (1973) Enzyme therapy in organic lesions of the spinal cord. Izdatelstvo akd nauk arm SSR Yerevan
107. Nicoll EA (1949) Fracture of the dorso-lumbar spine. J Bone Joint Surg 31 (3): 376 – 394
108. Nicoll EA (1962) Modern Trends in Orthopedics. 3: 100 – 129
109. Norrell H (1978) The treatment of unstable spinal fractures and dislocations. Clin Neurosurg 25: 193 – 208
110. Norrell H (1979) The early management of spinal injuries. Clin Neurosurg 27
111. Oganesian SS, Matinian LA (1964) Some clinical data on the enzyme therapy of spinal cord injuries. Tenth conf. I.P. Pavlov All. Union Physiol. Soc Yerevan 22: 213 – 214
112. Oganesian SS, Matinian LA, Meliksetian SA, Merzoian EG (1971) Certain problems of the treatment of trauma of the vertebral column and spinal cord. First all union congr Neurosurg (Moscow) 4: 179 – 183
113. O'Callaghan JP, Ullrich CG, Yvan HA, Kieffer SA (1980) CT of facet distraction in flexion injuries of the thoraco lumbar spine: the naked facet. AJR 134: 563 – 567
114. O'Laoire SA, Thomas, DGT (1982) Surgery in incomplete spinal cord injury. Surg Neurol 17 (1): 12 – 15
115. Osebold R, Weinstein SL, Sprague BL (1981) Thoraco-lumbar spine fractures. Results of treatment. Spine 6 (1): 13 – 34
116. Patil A (1981) Intercostal nerves to spinal nerve roots anastomosis (spinal cord bypass and Harrington rod fusion in traumatic paraplegia. Technical note. Acta Neurochir (Wien) 57 (3–4): 299 – 303
117. Paul RL, Michael RH, Dunn JE, Williams JP (1975) Anterior transthoracic surgical decompression of acute spinal cord injuries. J Neurosurg 43: 299 – 307
118. Peatfield RC *et al* (1983) Suprapubic catheterisation after spinal cord injury. A follow-up report. Paraplegia 21 (4): 220 – 226
119. Pennal GF (1966) Stress studies of the lumbar spine. Proceedings of the British orthopedics ass. J Bone Joint Surg 48 B: 180
120. Perves A, Pidhorz (1973) Fractures du rachis dorsal et lombaire. Indications opératoires et résultats. Rev Chir Orthop 59: 491 – 512
121. Pettegrew RK, Windle WF (1976) Factors in recovery from spinal cord injury. Exp Neurol 53: 815 – 829
122. Petter CK (1933) Methods of measuring the pressure of the intervertebral disc. J Bone Joint Surg 15: 365 – 368
123. Pierce DS (1969) Spinal cord injury with anterior decompression fusion and stabilization and early rehabilitation. J Bone Joint Surg 51 A: 1675
124. Rennie W, Mitchell N (1973) Flexion distraction fractures of the thoraco-lumbar spine. J Bone Joint Surg 55 A (2): 386 – 390
125. Rieunau G (1970) Manuel de traumatologie. 3e éd. Masson, Paris

126. Roaf R (1960) A study of the mechanics of spinal injuries. J Bone Joint Surg 42 B: 810–823
127. Roberts JB, Curtiss PH (1970) Stability of the thoracic and lumbar spine in traumatic paraplegia following fracture or fracture-dislocation. J Bone Joint Surg 52 A: 1115–1130
128. Rogers LF, Thayer C, Weinberg PE, Kwang SK (1980) Acute injuries of the upper thoracic spine associated with paraplegia. AJR 134: 67–73
129. Roy-Camille R, Berteaux D, Saillant J (1977) Synthèse du rachis dorso-lombaire traumatique par plaques vissées dans les pédicules vertébraux. Rev Chir Orthop 63: 452–456
130. Roy-Camille R et M, Demeulenaere (1970) Ostéosynthèse du rachis dorsal, lombaire et lombosacré per plaques métalliques vissées dans les pédicules vertébraux et les apophyses articulaires. Presse Méd 78 (32): 1447–1448
131. Roy-Camille R, Demeulenaere C, Barsat E, Saillant G (1973) Ostéosynthèse du rachis dorsal et lombaire par voie postérieure. Nouv Presse Méd 2 (19): 1309–1312
132. Roy-Camille R, Zerah JC (1970) Ostéosynthèse des fractures du rachis dorsal et lombaire. Act Chir Orthop de l'Hôpital Raymond Poincaré 8: 196–203
133. Saillant G (1976) Etude anatomique des pédicules vertébraux. Rev Chir Orthop 62: 151–160
134. Seljeskog EL (1982) Thoraco-lumbar injuries. Clin Neurosurg 30: 626–641
135. Schmidek HH, Gomes FB, Seligson D, Mc Sherry JW (1980) Management of acute unstable thoraco-lumbar (T 11 – L 1) fractures with and without neurological deficit. Neurosurgery 7 (1): 30–35
136. Schneider RC (1955) The syndrome of acute anterior spinal cord injury. J Neurosurg 12: 95–122
137. Schmorl G, Junghans M (1956) Clinique et radiologie de la colonne vertébrale normale et pathologique. Confrontation anatomopathologique. Trad JL Wolf-Fried G. Doin et Cie, Edit
138. Smith WS, Kaufer H, Arbor A (1969) Patterns and mechanisms of lumbar injuries associated with lap seat belts. JB JS 51 A (2): 239–254
139. Terver S (1975) Réflexions critiques sur le traitement des fractures graves du rachis dorso-lombaire par laminectomie ostéosynthèse. Thèse médecine Clermont-Ferrand
140. Vlahovitch B, Fuentes JM, Choucair Y, Blanchet P, Glatz E, Stoppa J (1978) Les fractures et luxations du rachis lombaire bas. J Chir 115 (12): 659–662
141. Vlahovitch B, Fuentes JM, Gary Bobo A, Bastian P, Facchini JP (1977) Justifications de quelques modifications apportées aux plaques de Roy Camille. Instantanées médicaux (EMC), Techniques Chirurgicales 5: 43–45
142. Watson-Jones R (1938) The results of postural reduction of fractures of the spine. J Bone Joint Surg (20): 567–586
143. Watson-Jones R (1949) Fractures of the spine. J Bone Joint Surg 31 B: 322–325
144. Watson-Jones R (1958) Fractures et lésions articulaires traumatiques. Adaptation française par J Roussel, Vol II. Delachaux et Niestlé, pp 989–1091

145. Wilson PD, Straub LR (1952) Arthrodèse vertébrale au moyen d'une plaque métallique. NY States J Med 52: 3003 – 3004
146. Whitesides TE Jr, Shah Sga (1976) On the management of unstable fractures of the thoraco-lumbar spine: rationale for use of anterior decompression and fusion and posterior stabilization. Spine 1: 99 – 107
147. Wrathall JR *et al* (1982) Reconstruction of the contused cat spinal cord by the delayed nerve graft technique and cultured peripheral non-neuronal cells. Acta Neuropathol (Berl) 57 (1): 59 – 69
148. Yeo JD, Lowry C, McKenzie B (1978): Preliminary report on ten patients with spinal cord injuries treated with hyperbaric oxygen. Med J Aust 2 (12): 572 – 573
149. Young B, Brooks WH, Tibbs PA (1981) Anterior decompression and fusion for thoraco lumbar fractures with neurological deficits. Acta Neurochir (Wien) 57: 287 – 298
150. Young JS, Dexter WR (1978) Neurological recovery distal to the zone of injury in 172 cases of closed, traumatic spinal cord injury. Paraplegia 16: 39 – 489
151. Young TD, Leatherman KD, Brown TD (1970) The early rod fixation in treatment of fracture-dislocation of the spine. Proceeding of the Am Acad of Orthopedic Surgeon. J Bone Joint Surg 52 A (6): 1257

# Non-operative Treatment—Rehabilitation and Outcome

H. L. Frankel[1], W. S. El Masri[2], and G. Ravichandran[3]

[1] National Spinal Injuries Centre, Stoke Mandeville Hospital, Aylesbury, Bucks (England),
[2] The Midland Spinal Injuries Centre, Institute of Orthopaedics, Oswestry, Shropshire (England),
[3] Spinal Injuries Unit, Lodge Moor Hospital, Sheffield (England)

With 12 Figures

## Contents

## 1. Introduction

*Scope of Chapter*

This chapter is confined to consideration of closed spinal cord and cauda equina injuries.

*Non-operative Treatment*

The indications and techniques of various early surgical procedures are described in other chapters. We shall concentrate on describing our routine practice of non-surgical treatment. In addition we will briefly mention those circumstances under which we would currently recommend early or delayed surgical procedures on the spine.

## 2. Management of Spinal Column Injury

In general this is achieved by postural reduction with pillows. Originally at Stoke Mandeville we used beds made of sorbo packs and the patients were turned regularly by manual turning. Nowadays we use a Stoke Mandeville Egerton turning bed, Figs. 1 and 2. This is an electrically controlled turning bed and it is possible to turn a patient without disturbing the attitude of his spine. It is however a normal practice to lift the patient with a full lifting team once in every twenty-four hours. On this occasion he is turned fully on his side for bowel care and for physiotherapy to the upper hip. The majority of fractures and fracture dislocations can be partially or completely reduced by this method. Pain relief is usually achieved early and it is possible to dispense with strong analgesics after two or three days.

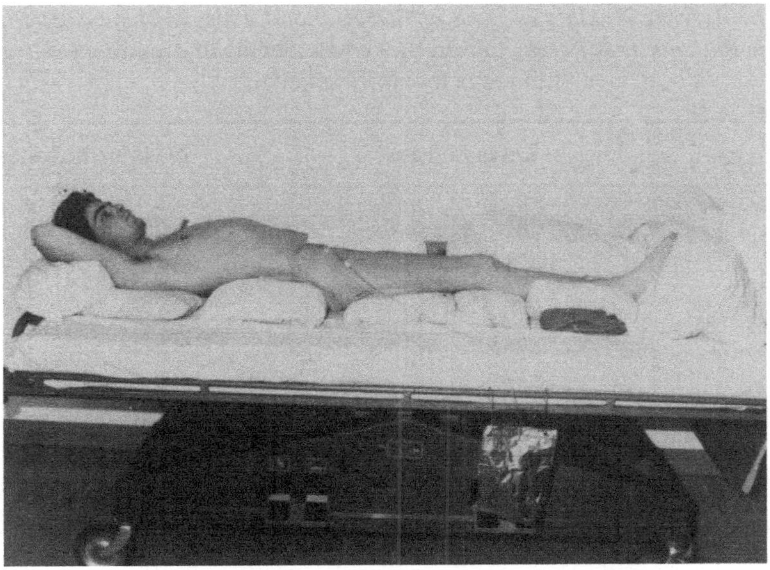

Fig. 1. Stoke Mandeville Egerton turning bed with patient on back

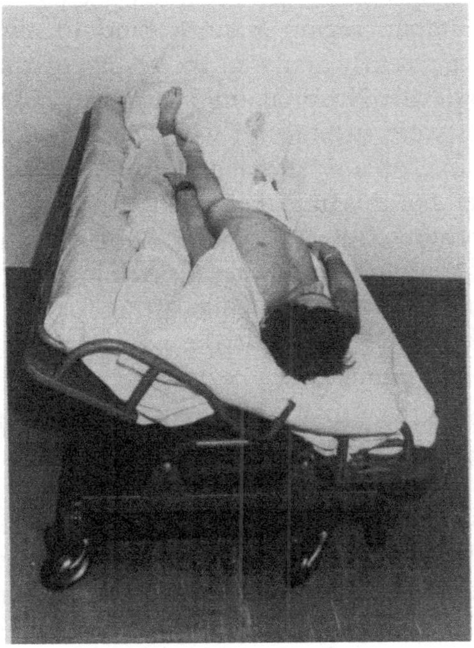

Fig. 2. Stoke Mandeville Egerton turning bed with patient tilted on side

Table 1. *The Average Number of Days of Bed Rest and Average Number of Days in Hospital for Patients at Different Levels.* Stoke Mandeville figures above, Oswestry figures below in brackets

| | Days bed rest | Days in hospital |
|---|---|---|
| D 1–D 6 | 49<br>(51) | 192<br>(145) |
| D 7–D 10 | 62.5<br>(54) | 177<br>(151) |
| D 11–L 1 | 77<br>(58) | 182<br>(139) |
| Below L 1 | 89<br>(63) | 170<br>(127) |

The length of time required for stability of the spine is variable but in general patients with injuries in the upper dorsal spine require six or seven weeks immobilization. Patients with injuries in the D 7 to D 10 region require approximately eight weeks immobilization and patients with injuries in the dorso-lumbar and lumbar region require nine to twelve weeks immobilization. We have recently analysed the results of a series of patients treated at Stoke Mandeville Hospital and at Oswestry. The period of bed rest until the patients were sitting in a wheelchair and length of stay in hospital are shown in Table 1 (Ravichandran, El Masri, Frankel—in preparation). At the end of this time the patients are transferred to a bed in which they can be progressively sat up and soon after learn to sit in a wheelchair. Patients with dorso-lumbar and lumbar injuries wear an anterior body vest to prevent flexion while sitting for the next few weeks. During the last two weeks of bed rest the patients practise exercises to strengthen their spinal musculature.

As an alternative to the Stoke Mandeville Egerton turning bed it is possible to manually turn the patient by lifting or log rolling. This is satisfactory if there is a team skilled in these methods. Alternatively, a Stryker frame can be used. Again this has proved satisfactory to those skilled in its use. There are considerable problems with the prone position in patients with higher lesions. In addition, the prone position in an extended spine gives rise to a degree of compression of the bony injury which is not present in the supine position where the weight of the body over the extending pillow causes a certain degree of traction. The circo-electric bed is, in our opinion, unsuitable for patients with unstable spines and may, in addition, cause severe transient postural hypotension in the acute stage.

### 3. Circumstances Under Which Non-operative Management is Inappropriate

1. Delayed onset of neurological deficit or increased density of neurological deficit. Under these circumstances appropriate neuro-radiological investigations must be performed urgently and, where appropriate, surgical intervention is indicated.
2. Inability of patient to co-operate with conservative treatment. This may occur in the case of mental deficiency, psychosis or delirium tremens.
3. Gross bony displacement which does not respond to conservative management within the first few days.
4. Cases where it is demonstrated that there is established instability of a dislocation. If Stoke Mandeville Egerton turning beds are available and/or there is adequate, specialized nursing care, surgical stabilization can be delayed in order to see whether spontaneous stability develops. In circumstances where special beds or skilled care are not available, a decision to stabilize the spine surgically must be taken at an early stage.

The presence of bony or disc fragments within the spinal canal does not necessarily constitute an indication for surgical intervention.

### 4. Neurological Outcome

The authors have only slight experience of examining patients within the first few hours after injury. What happens both clinically and pathologically during these early hours is naturally of great interest and potential importance. As far as we can ascertain from the clinical point of view, in most cases the maximal neurological deficit is immediately after injury. It is not unusual for a spinal cord lesion to ascend by one or two segments within the first few days and this is almost always followed by recovery to the original or a slightly lower level. Rarely, a more serious form of ascending lesion occurs (Frankel 1969). These cases usually become apparent between the 2nd and 11th day following injury and the lesion ascends segment by segment for a number of days. There is usually associated pyrexia and severe pain in those segments which are about to be lost. Ascending lesions are most common in patients with dorso-lumbar lesions and one case rose from L 4 segment to C 8 segment. The incidence of this phenomenon in dorso-lumbar lesions is between 1.5% and 2%. The aetiology of these cases is probably not always the same and extrinsic compression by haematoma must obviously be excluded. Although ascending thrombosis and ascending haematomyelia are possible aetiologies, we believe that the majority are due to an inflammatory or necrotising lesion which might be called "Ascending Myelitis". It is reasonable to treat such patients with systemic cortico-steroids once the lesion has ascended more than two segments. We do not use routine cortico-steroids in patients with traumatic spinal cord lesions as we have found no evidence that they are beneficial.

### 4.1. Systems of Neurological Classification

There is, as yet, no entirely satisfactory method of documenting neurological progression in spinal cord injuries. Many publications have used terms such as "complete", "virtually complete", "incomplete" and "improved" without further definition. The system devised at Stoke Mandeville Hospital (Frankel *et al.* 1969) is easy to use and is probably the most sophisticated system that is useful for large scale, retrospective studies. It is most suited to spinal cord lesions and its accuracy and utility diminishes in cauda equina lesions as the system cannot accommodate changes of level. It is, however, a system that is useful in comparing patients initial and final neurological status. The system is as follows:

A. *Complete.* This means that the lesion is found to be complete, both motor and sensory, below the segmental level named.

B. *Sensory incompleteness only.* This implies that there is some sensation present below the level of the lesion but that the motor paralysis is complete below that level. This does not apply when there is slight discrepancy between motor and sensory level but does apply to "sacral sparing".

C. *Motor useless.* This implies that there is some motor power present below the lesion but it is of no practical use to the patient.

D. *Motor useful.* This implies that there is useful motor power below the level of the lesion. Patients in this group can move the lower limbs and many can walk with or without aids.

E. *Recovery.* This implies that the patient is free of neurological symptoms, i.e., no weakness, no sensory loss, no sphincter disturbance. Abnormal reflexes may be present.

A somewhat similar system with more emphasis on sensory function was introduced by Bohlman (1979) and modified by Bohlman, Freehafer and Dejak (1985). For prospective studies a more sophisticated classification can be used such as the Yale Index (Bracken, Webb and Wagner 1978, Chehrazi *et al.* 1981) but this requires a high standard of examination and documentation.

### 4.2. Expected Neurological Evolution at Different Spinal Levels

Frankel *et al.* (1969) separated their patients by level of the spinal column injury into groups, D 1–D 10, D 11, D 12, and L 1 (dorso-lumbar) and lumbar injuries. The D 1–D 10 group had a higher percentage of initially complete lesions (81%) than the dorso-lumbar cases (61%). There was proportionately a greater degree of improvement by at least one grade in the dorso-lumbar group. The number of lumbar cases was too small for meaningful analysis.

In the series of Frankel *et al.* (1969) all of the patients were treated by non-operative means and an attempt was made to correlate the severity of fracture dislocation and the degree of reduction achieved with the neurological outcome. At all levels the grossly displaced fracture dislocations had a higher percentage of complete lesions, both initially and on discharge. However, in the lesser dislocations, the degree of reduction achieved did not seem to influence the end result.

Young and Dexter (1978) analysed a series of patients using similar entry criteria and the same method of classification. 26% of their D 1–D 10 cases and 60% of their dorso-lumbar cases had had laminectomies, 62.6% had received Dexamethasone. According to their analysis there was no significant difference between the neurological progression of their patients and those reported in the earlier Stoke Mandeville study. There are, however, great difficulties in statistical evaluation of results based on a ranking system such as the Frankel classification. However, by inspection of the published data of Young and Dexter it is apparent that the natural history of spinal cord lesions is similarly revealed by both Centres. Bohlman, Freehafer and Dejak (1985) reported that of 149 patients with injuries to the upper thoracic spine (defined by them as D 1–D 10) who had complete lesions on admission to their Service, none recovered any significant neurological function regardless of the type of operative or non-operative treatment. This has had marked variance with the results from Stoke Mandeville and Phoenix and is perhaps attributable to the fact that patients were only considered to have a complete lesion if they had "total motor and sensory loss below the level of the bony injury that lasted for more than 48 hours after admission". The Stoke Mandeville and Phoenix studies had accepted the first reliable examination in their own Centres as the entry point and in many cases this was within the first 24 hours.

Burke, Burley and Ungar (1985) reporting from Melbourne, Australia had similar results to the original Stoke Mandeville series but did not differentiate between different levels. Wilmot and Hall (1986) described 95 paraplegics, their level not being further defined. They found no improvement in any patients admitted to their study with a complete lesion. They attempted to compare those patients who had had surgical stabilization with those who had had no surgery and they concluded that "complications were significantly greater in patients who underwent internal fixation surgery. The neurological condition did not appear to be jeopardized by rodding and fusion". The patients had not been selected for operative or conservative management by a random process.

We are currently comparing a group of patients treated at Stoke Mandeville with a similar group treated at Oswestry (El Masri, Ravichandran and Frankel—in preparation). In order to discover whether there was any difference between those with skeletal injuries at D 1–D 6 and D 7–D 10, we analysed these separately. Dorso-lumbar and lumbar cases were grouped as previously. The results are shown in Tables 2, 3, 4, and 5.

Table 2. *D 1–D 6*. In the squares in the grid are two letters, the first relates to the neurological lesion on admission and the second to the neurological lesion on discharge. The upper figures are for Stoke Mandeville cases and the lower figures in brackets refer to Oswestry cases

| | | | | |
|---|---|---|---|---|
| AA<br>19<br>(19) | AB<br>1<br>(1) | AC<br>3<br>(1) | AD | AE |
| BA | BB<br>3<br>(2) | BC<br>1 | BD<br>4<br>(1) | BE<br>2 |
| CA<br>(1) | CB | CC | CD<br>2<br>(1) | CE<br>(1) |
| DA | DB | DC | DD | DE<br>(2) |
| EA | EB | EC | ED | EE<br>(1) |

Table 3. *D 7–D 10*. In the squares in the grid are two letters, the first relates to the neurological lesion on admission and the second to the neurological lesion on discharge. The upper figures are for Stoke Mandeville cases and the lower figures in brackets refer to Oswestry cases

| | | | | |
|---|---|---|---|---|
| AA<br>17<br>(13) | AB<br>3 | AC<br>1 | AD<br>1 | AE |
| BA | BB | BC | BD | BE |
| CA | CB | CC | CD<br>1<br>(1) | CE<br>(1) |
| DA | DB | DC | DD | DE |
| EA | EB | EC | ED | EE |

Table 4. *D 11–L 1.* In the squares in the grid are two letters, the first relates to the neurological lesion on admission and the second to the neurological lesion on discharge. The upper figures are for Stoke Mandeville cases and the lower figures in brackets refer to Oswestry cases

| | | | | |
|---|---|---|---|---|
| AA<br>28<br>(19) | AB<br>1<br>(1) | AC<br>6<br>(3) | AD<br>1<br>(3) | AE<br><br>(1) |
| BA<br>1 | BB<br>1<br>(3) | BC<br>1<br>(1) | BD<br>5 | BE |
| CA<br>1 | CB | CC<br>5 | CD<br>5<br>(7) | CE<br>2<br>(2) |
| DA | DB | DC | DD<br>2<br>(3) | DE<br>2<br>(4) |
| EA | EB | EC | ED | EE<br><br>(3) |

Table 5. *Below L 1.* In the squares in the grid are two letters, the first relates to the neurological lesion on admission and the second to the neurological lesion on discharge. The upper figures are for Stoke Mandeville cases and the lower figures in brackets refer to Oswestry cases

| | | | | |
|---|---|---|---|---|
| AA<br>2 | AB<br><br>(1) | AC<br>1<br>(1) | AD<br>1<br>(1) | AE |
| BA | BB<br>1<br>(1) | BC<br>2 | BD<br>1<br>(1) | BE |
| CA | CB | CC<br>2<br>(1) | CD<br><br>(2) | CE<br>2<br>(1) |
| DA | DB | DC | DD<br>1 | DE<br><br>(4) |
| EA | EB | EC | ED | EE<br><br>(2) |

Somewhat surprisingly we found a high proportion (92%) of patients with initially complete lesions in the D 7–D 10 group. In the D 1–D 6 group only 67% had initially complete lesions. Taking the combined groups of D 1–D 6 and D 7–D 10, the percentage of those with initially complete lesions was 76% which does not differ significantly from the 1969 Stoke Mandeville series (81%). The dorso-lumbar group—56% initially complete, approximates closely to the original Stoke Mandeville series (61%).

The few papers mentioned above demonstrate discrepancies between those Centres that found a small but significant number of patients who improved after having sustained clinically complete spinal cord lesions and those who found no such cases. However, the results from Stoke Mandeville, Oswestry, Phoenix and Melbourne, demonstrate that a small but important percentage of patients who have such an initial, complete lesion, did make a significant improvement. All the authors agree that in initially incomplete cases there is a greater possibility of further improvement. In order for future studies of different forms of initial therapy to be conducted successfully and ethically, it will be necessary to use a unified method of examination and classification and also to have fixed entry times to these studies.

## 5. Management of Different Systems and Problems During Bed Rest and During Period of Active Rehabilitation

A patient with a complete spinal cord lesion is prone to many disturbances and complications, these are all direct or indirect results of the disordered physiology resulting from the spinal cord lesion. Individually or together these may be expected to lead to the early death of the patient unless they are understood and controlled. The major complications that may be expected are:

a) Respiratory complications
b) Gastro-intestinal complications
c) Cardiovascular complications and problems
d) Urinary tract complications
e) Pressure sores
f) Contractures
g) Problems related to associated injuries
h) Spacticity
i) Pain

a) *Respiratory complications* are most common in patients with upper or mid dorsal injuries. However, complications arise, both as a result of direct injuries to the thorax and due to paralysis of intercostal muscles and abdominal muscles. Spinal fractures require a regime of nursing which may make it difficult to obtain adequate X-rays and any therapy that is required must conform to the required nursing position. In addition to routine management of chest injuries the patients require skilled physiotherapy to assist them with coughing.

During the later stages these problems are rarely very serious in paraplegics. However, those with higher lesions have a life long impairment of coughing.

b) *Gastro-intestinal complications.* Patients with upper dorsal cord lesions often develop a partial neurogenic ileus. This may only become fully apparent after two or three days. It is important that the patients receive only limited amounts of clear fluids by mouth in the first few days. If a fully developed ileus and gastric dilatation develops, the patient will need to be treated by "drip and suck" until the condition has resolved.

Patients with dorso-lumbar or lumbar injuries often have substantial retro-peritoneal haematoma. The ensuing rigidity and distension of the abdomen may be difficult to distinguish from intra-peritoneal injuries.

Bleeding into the stomach or duodenum from acute stress ulcers is an occasional complication. This bleeding usually occurs in the first few days. Fibre optic endoscopy can usually make an accurate diagnosis and the appropriate treatment can be given. The authors do not currently use routine prophylactic H 2 blockers.

In the chronic stage there are very rarely any problems with gastric or intestinal function. However, if the patients are subjected to a new stress such as an anaesthetic with or without operation, then they may again have a temporary period of ileus.

Bowel function is seriously impaired in complete paraplegics but can usually be successfully regulated by artificial means (Frankel 1967). We usually recommend a mild laxative such as Senna on alternate afternoons or evenings (the exact dose and timing is a matter of individual variation). The following morning two glycerine suppositories are inserted into the rectum. This should cause reflex defecation in patients with upper motor neurone lesions. This reflex defecation may be efficient but the patients also know how to perform gentle, digital evacuations. Patients with lower motor neurone lesions can rarely empty the rectum completely by straining and attempts to do so may cause pseudo-prolapse of the rectum. They, therefore, usually perform digital evacuations on themselves. Even patients with complete lesions can usually learn to avoid "bowel accidents". Patients with incomplete lesions usually regain some bowel sensation and control but they still have a marked tendency to become constipated and severe constipation can lead to spurious diarrhoea.

c) *Cardiovascular complications and problems.* Venous thrombosis and pulmonary emboli are relatively common, Walsh and Tribe (1965), Watson (1978), Perkash (1978) and El Masri and Silver (1981). Unless there is a contra-indication to anticoagulation, the authors routinely use oral anticoagulation with Phenindione or Warfarin, starting at about the fifth day after injury. The majority of fatal pulmonary emboli occur between the tenth and thirtieth day after injury, and by means of oral anticoagulation, this mortality can be avoided. In patients with associated injuries or a medical history that precludes the use of oral anticoagulation we either give no anticoagulant at all, or alternatively use low or medium dose subcutaneous Heparin.

During the phase of bed rest the most common problem is of venous thrombosis and thrombo embolism which are common in the early weeks after spinal cord injury, they are virtually unknown in the chronic stage (Frankel and Mathias 1976).

## Postural Hypotension

The resting blood pressure in patients with upper dorsal lesions is low (Frankel *et al.* 1972). When patients first sit up following a period of bed rest they often suffer from severe postural hypotension. They learn to sit up by an arbitrary system of training. This first consists of sitting the patient up slightly in a winding bed. This process is repeated several times each day. Later the patient sits in a wheelchair, first for a few minutes and then for longer periods. Soon all patients can tolerate the sitting position for long periods. The mechanism by which the arbitrary training is mediated is partly by activation of the renin angiotensin system and by the release of vasopressin. It is important that patients with incomplete lesions should not be subjected to severe hypotension when first mobilized as this may cause a temporary deterioration in their neurological state (El Masri and Baker—submitted for publication).

## Autonomic Dysreflexia

The phenomenon occurs in its major form only in patients with high spinal cord lesions. Autonomic dysreflexia is precipitated by bladder contractions, rectal contractions, ejaculation, contraction of the pregnant uterus, skeletal muscle spasms and any phenomenon in the paralysed part of the body which in the intact person would cause severe pain, e.g., squeezing an infected, ingrowing toe nail. There is intense vasoconstriction of resistance and capacitance vessels below the level of the lesion and this results in severe hypertension. In patients with complete lesions below D 1 and D 2 there is often a reflex bradycardia, in patients with slightly lower lesions there may be bradycardia or tachycardia and dysrhythmias are common. In severe, unrelieved cases there may be severe throbbing headaches and occasionally hypertensive encephalopathy or cerebral haemorrhage.

The management of autonomic dysreflexia is by identifying and removing the cause. In an emergency the blood pressure may be reduced by the use of drugs such as locally applied lignocaine, drugs acting at the level of the isolated spinal cord (clonidine, reserpine or spinal anaesthetics), drugs acting on the ganglia (hexamethonium), drugs acting on the sympathetic nerve terminals (guanethidine) or directly on the blood vessels (glyceryl trinitrate). Glyceryl trinitrate is the most easily managed drug and the patients may administer it themselves either in the form of sub-lingual tablets (maximum dose 300 microgrammes) or trans-dermally.

Autonomic dysreflexia is a very important warning symptom in patients with a high spinal cord lesion and failure to recognize it and rectify the cause may have serious consequences. For a fuller account of this phenomenon see Frankel and Mathias (1979) and for an account of other autonomic problems in spinal cord injuries see Mathias and Frankel (1983).

d) *Urinary tract complications.* In the first days after spinal cord lesion, whether it is complete or incomplete, there is usually a period of complete retention of urine. This is almost always managed by some form of catheterization. The methods currently most often used are

i. intermittent catheterization
ii. indwelling urethral catheterization
iii. a fine bore supra-pubic catheterization.

Each of these methods has its advantages and disadvantages. Outside specialized spinal injuries units, it is most common to use an indwelling urethral catheter of the Foley type. The most common complications of that form of catheterization are urinary tract infections, urethral diverticuli and fistulae and epididymo orchitis. These complications can be reduced by correct positioning of the catheter and by regular changes of the catheter.

Whatever method of bladder management is adopted, urinary tract complications remain a significant source of morbidity to paraplegic patients. For this reason patients need to remain under the care of their spinal injuries unit for the rest of their lives. Many patients will ultimately develop reflex "automatic bladders" and some will have bladders that can be expressed by manual pressure or abdominal straining. In the opinion of the authors the primary objective is to obtain adequate bladder emptying without the use of catheters and if possible the patients should have sterile urine. Even if this state can be achieved, regular urological review is still necessary in order to detect those patients who develop upper urinary tract dilatation and other complications. In order to achieve this catheter free state, a small proportion of the male patients require surgery to the bladder neck and/or external sphincter. Almost all male patients with complete lesions treated in this way need to use an external urinal device such as a condom urinal.

Some patients cannot achieve adequate voiding. In the past these were usually treated with long term indwelling catheters, usually urethral but occasionally supra-pubic. Although this is not the first choice of treatment, if carefully managed with a high fluid intake, this method is compatible with long term survival.

More recently the method of long term intermittent self catheterization has been reintroduced for both male and female patients. The long term results of this method have not yet been evaluated.

The situation of female paraplegics if far less satisfactory as no functional female urinal has yet been developed. Traditionally female patients have been taught to stimulate their bladder to empty either by tapping or straining before it empties itself. In many cases this has been unsatisfactory and those patients have either resorted to the use of long term indwelling catheters or have been chronically wet. Recently, electrical stimulation of selected anterior sacral nerve roots has been introduced by Professor Giles Brindley (Cardozo *et al.* 1984). This procedure combined with the surgical division of some posterior sacral roots, has given functional continence to some of the female patients. Electrical stimulation of anterior sacral nerve roots has also been used in male patients.

e) *Pressure sores* are bound to develop unless the patient is turned regularly. On a Stoke Mandeville Egerton turning bed this is performed every three hours. If patients are turned on other turning beds or manually, they must also be turned to a new position every three hours. In addition, the pressure points must be examined daily. By these means, it is possible to totally prevent pressure sores in the acute stages. It is a regrettable fact that spinal injuries centres still receive a certain number of patients who have already developed significant pressure sores in the first days after injury. The tendency to develop pressure sores is a long term one. Therefore, the patients must learn to lift themselves every 15 minutes while sitting in the wheelchair and to turn themselves regularly while in bed. The frequency of turning while in bed is a matter of trial and error. In the first instance the patients turn themselves every 3 hours and then gradually extend that period to a maximum of 6 hours. In addition, the patients learn to inspect their pressure areas daily and if there is the slightest redness or bruising they must keep off that part until the condition has resolved. By these means the majority of patients remain free of pressure sores but a small proportion of ex-patients develop severe pressure sores which may be life threatening and may occasionally lead to secondary amyloidosis. In patients who develop recurrent pressure sores there is usually a psychological or social cause.

f) *Contractures.* There is a great tendency for soft tissue contractures around paralysed joints to develop. This tendency is most marked in the first few weeks after the onset of paralysis. The patients need to be nursed in a position that will minimize the tendency towards contractures. In addition, they require a full range of passive movements to all paralysed joints twice a day, seven days a week.

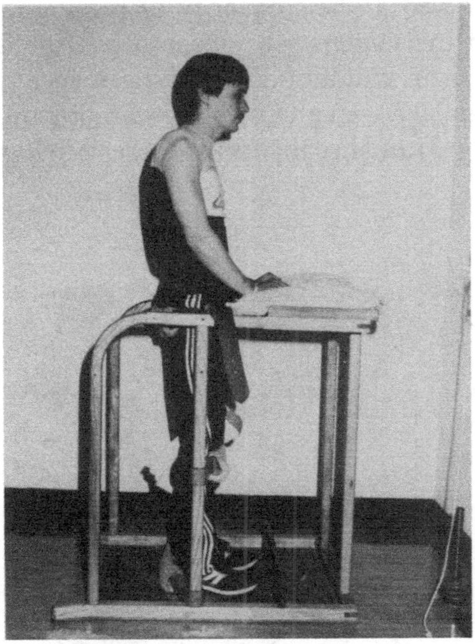

Fig. 3. Oswestry standing frame

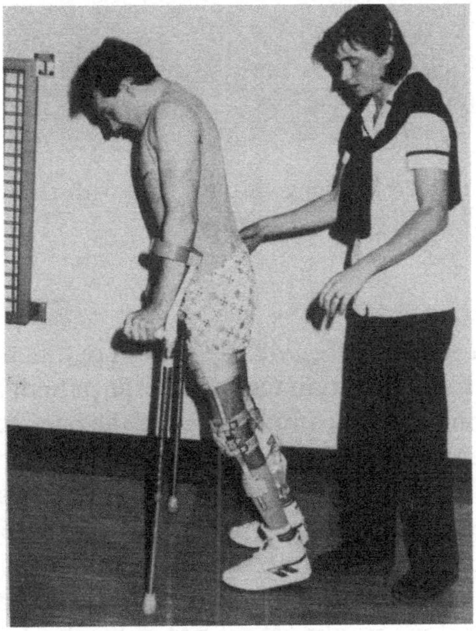

Fig. 4. Patient being trained to ambulate with elbow crutches and long calipers

After the first six weeks, the frequency of passive movements can be reduced. In children the tendency to develop contractures remains very strong throughout their childhood and adolescence. Patients are encouraged to stand regularly—in an Oswestry standing frame for those with lesions above D 9 (Fig. 3) and in calipers for those with lower lesions (Figs. 4 and 5).

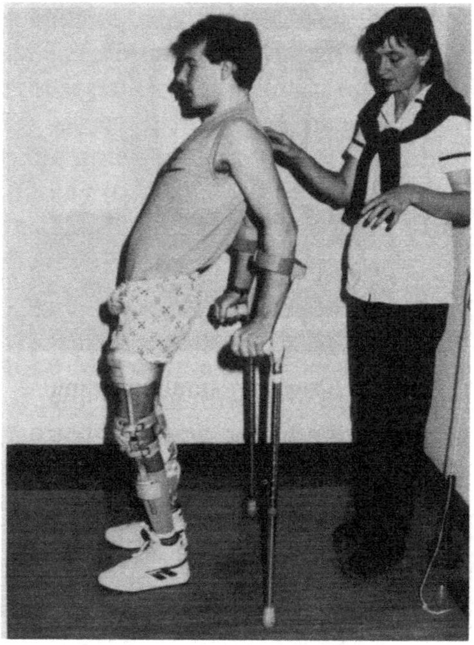

Fig. 5. Patient being trained in swing through gait with elbow crutches and long calipers

g) *Problems related to associated injuries.* Treatment of these injuries must be fitted into the overall management of the patient and fractures must be treated in anticipation of the importance of the particular limb involved. For example, upper limb fractures are treated by internal fixation more frequently than in non-paralysed patients, as the posture required for conservative management of these fractures is often not available. Operative procedures on fractured limbs should, whenever possible, be done early so that routine anticoagulation can start at the appropriate time.

h) *Spasticity* develops in almost all patients who have any remaining isolated spinal cord. This is not only to be expected, it brings with it certain benefits such as maintaining circulation, reducing wasting, reducing susceptibility to pressure sores and lessening of the demineralization of the bones of the spine, pelvis and lower limbs. Patients with complete cord lesions who have been well managed from the outset, rarely have disabling spasticity. Patients with slightly incomplete lesions often have the most intractable spasticity. In such cases the first line of approach should be by adequate, proper positioning and passive movements and the use of a standing frame. Hydrotherapy in a warm pool and local cooling with ice may be beneficial. Drug treatment should, if possible, be avoided. The drugs in common use are Diazepam, Baclofen and Dantrolene sodium. Peripheral surgical procedures on tendons may help, in particular division of the hamstring tendons and lengthening of the Achilles tendons. Surgical anterior rhizotomy is known to give permanent relief of spasticity but because of the number of roots required, is rarely performed. Posterior rhizotomy by chemicals or radio frequency probe, at several levels, often gives relief but the effect may not be permanent. Injection of 6% Phenol in water into motor points may be successful. Intrathecal alcohol will certainly abolish all spasticity but the price to be paid in terms of bladder and bowel function and severe wasting is very high.

Patients who have developed a set pattern and degree of spasticity and who after some years of stability develop a different pattern or an increase in spasticity, should be investigated for some underlying pathology in the anaesthetic parts of their bodies.

i) *Pain*. Fortunately most patients with paraplegia due to closed spinal injuries do not suffer any pain. Some patients do have pain and this may be in the nature of phantom pains, root pains or hyperpathic pains. Phantom pains can usually be avoided by early, active rehabilitation. At the earliest sign of their appearance the phantom nature of their pains should be explained to the patient. This, together with diversional therapy, usually reduces the phenomenon to an acceptable level. Occasionally psychotherapy is helpful. Drug treatment with large doses of Carbamazepine combined with anti-depressants are often prescribed and appear to be effective in some cases. Root pains which occur immediately below the last innervated segment are rare but particularly difficult to treat. Again, diversional therapy is the most likely to succeed. In severe cases, cordotomy and even cordectomy just above the lesion have been tried. The procedures sometimes give relief, unfortunately, the relief is usually temporary. Neurosurgically produced lesions in the dorsal root entry zone above the traumatic spinal cord lesion, are being evaluated.

Symptoms on the border line of the neurological lesion where partial or abnormal sensation is present, can be particularly troublesome as the patient may not be able to bear the slightest touch in that place. In these cases a surgically or chemically induced lesion of the appropriate peripheral nerve will give relief.

## 6. Physical Rehabilitation

During the period of bed rest the patient receives regular passive movements to the paralysed joints and systematic muscle strengthening exercises to the normal musculature. Once a patient is sitting in the wheelchair he must achieve adequate sitting balance. This is taught in the

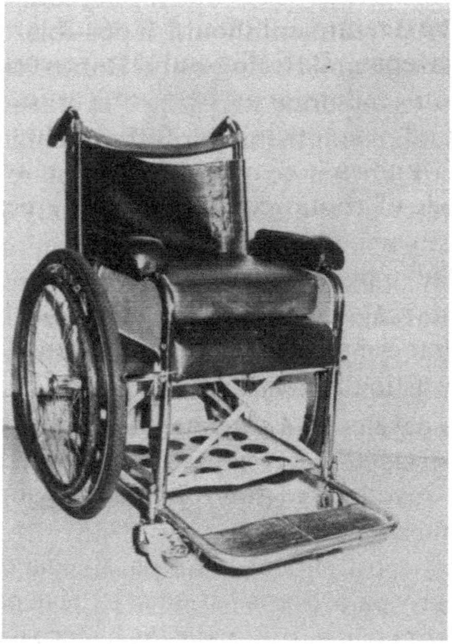

Fig. 6. Wheelchair dating from 2nd World War

first instance in front of a mirror and when this is satisfactory, with the eyes shut.

The patients then learn good wheelchair control and the majority of paraplegics can learn "back wheel balance" for mounting kerbs. Almost all paraplegics are capable of learning independent transfers from bed-chair-bed, chair-toilet-chair, chair-car-chair and many patients can also learn floor to chair transfers.

During the period of rehabilitation which is relatively long at Stoke Mandeville and Oswestry and rather short in some other centres such as the Santa Clara Valley Medical Centre (Wilmot and Hall 1986), the patients should become fully independent in their activities of daily living. They should learn to drive a suitably adapted hand controlled car. Patients with lesions below D 9 can often learn to ambulate effectively with the aid of long calipers and elbow crutches (Figs. 4 and 5). In some cases this will be a useful means of ambulation but the majority of patients with lesions above L 1 are

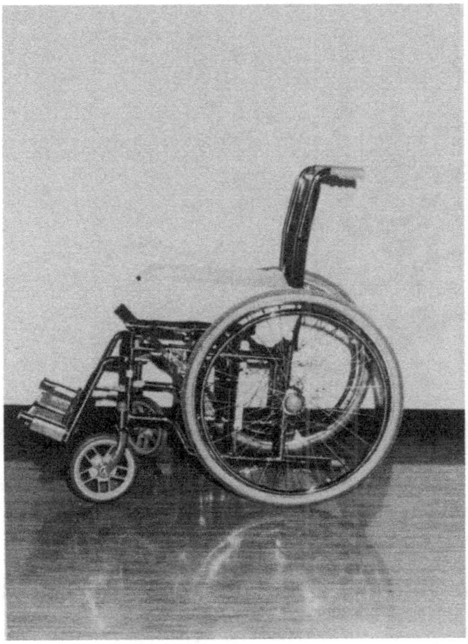

Fig. 7. Wheelchair of the classical Everest & Jennings type

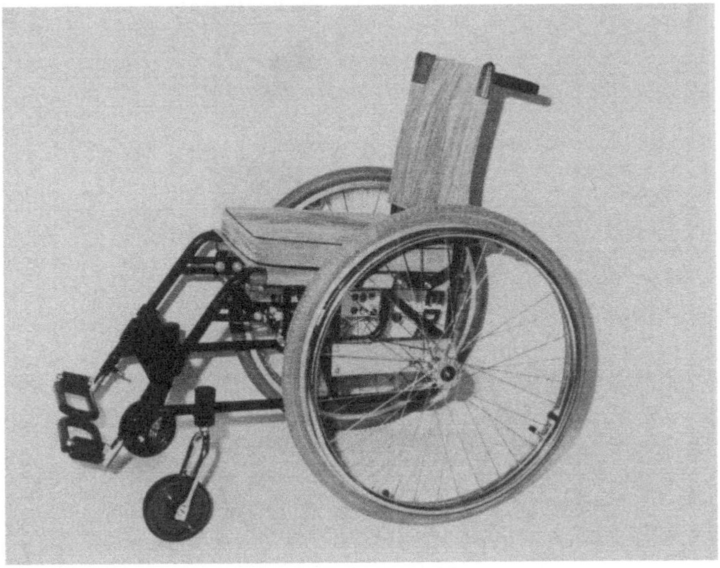

Fig. 8. Modern lightweight wheelchair

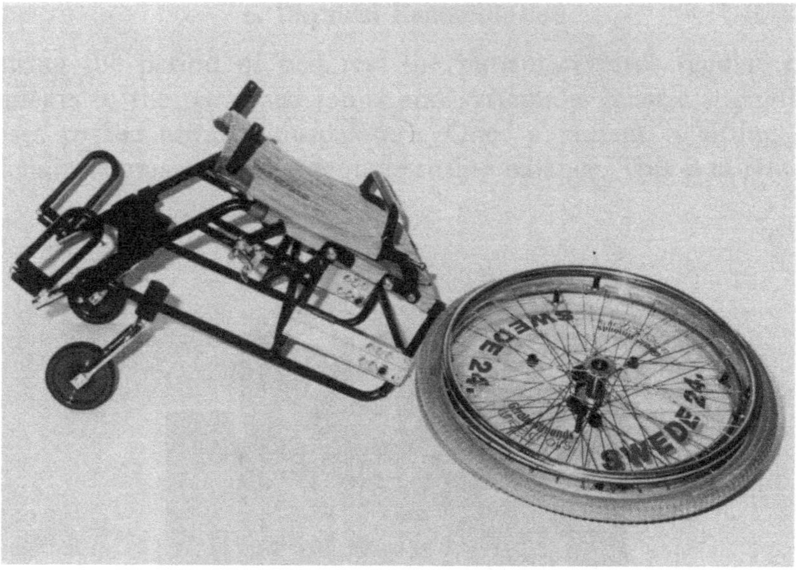


Fig. 9. Modern lightweight wheelchair with wheels removed from frame

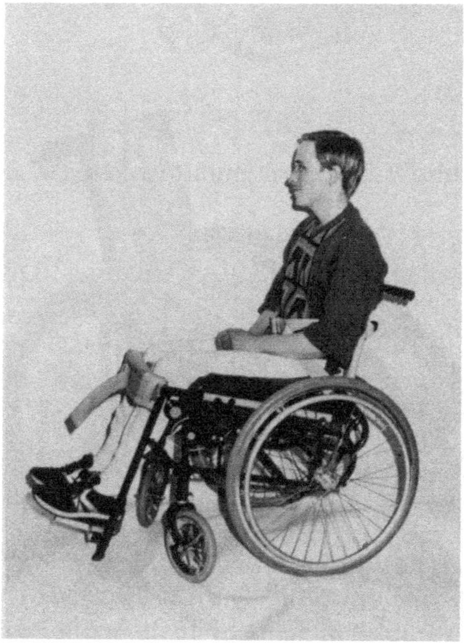

Fig. 10. The Levo active wheelchair in sitting position

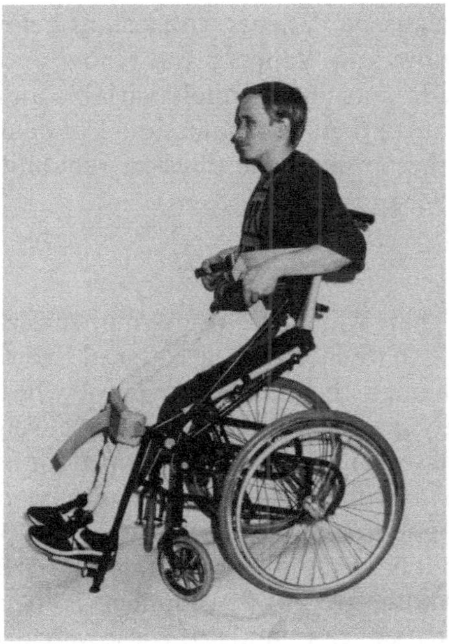

Fig. 11. The Levo active wheelchair in half up position

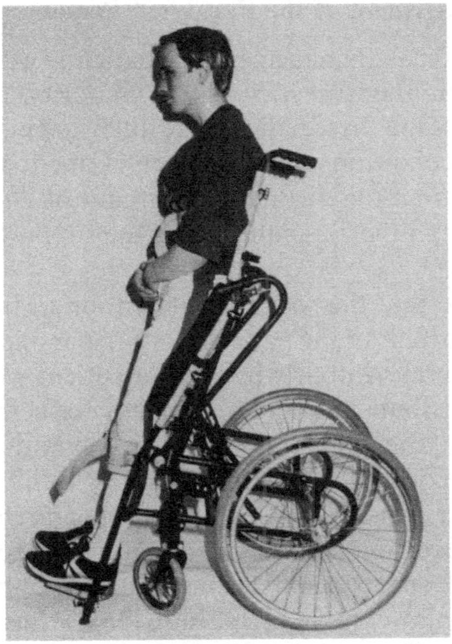

Fig. 12. The Levo active wheelchair in standing position

still substantial wheelchair users. Patients with lesions below L 3 can often walk with the aid of below knee calipers and elbow crutches or sticks. Patients with incomplete lesions are infinitely variable and their function depends on the exact nature of their residual lesion. For details of the actual techniques used by the therapists in the physical rehabilitation of spinal patients, see Bromley (1985).

### *6.1. Wheelchairs*

The traditional wheelchair which was in use immediately after the 2nd World War (Fig. 6) was soon replaced by the classical Everest and Jennings design (Fig. 7). This remained the standard type of wheelchair for over thirty years. More recently specialized, adjustable, light weight wheelchairs have been introduced. These were originally developed for use in wheelchair sport but their lightness and manoeuvrability and ease of control have rendered them extremely popular with the majority of paraplegics. Many of these chairs do not fold but have rapidly removable wheels for transporting in cars (Figs. 8 and 9). Another recent development is the introduction of wheelchairs in which the patient can stand up. These were originally worked by a battery powered electrical motor which rendered them heavy and bulky. The most recent model is manually operated and is an effective and manoeuvrable wheelchair in its own right (Figs. 10, 11, and 12).

## 7. Management of the Paralysed Person

Advances in the medical management of patients with spinal cord injuries have resulted in the survival of the majority to a long life expectancy. The quality of life these patients are likely to enjoy depends not only on their medical condition and their achievement of a good rehabilitation state but also on the quality and amount of effort directed at their social re-integration in the community and the support and guidance on pscho-sexual matters.

It must be appreciated that the social re-integration of the patient with spinal cord injury is important to the patient, his partner and family as well as the community in general. A poorly integrated patient withdrawn from society is unlikely to contribute to it and more likely to further draw on its resources. The majority of these patients have their injury during the active period of their life while contributing with their work to the welfare of the society they live in; their reward being financial and hierarchical providing them with a sense of achievement. Most individuals in this age group take an active part in one or more sports and have one or more hobbies which they not only enjoy but also enjoy competing in. Individuals thus form ties with partners, relatives, friends, the local community and to varying degrees with the society in general.

The problems patients who sustain a spinal cord injury have to contend with can be summarized as follows:

1. Varying degrees of paralysis of the locomotor system according to the level and the extent of the lesion in the transverse and longitudinal plane. This results in varying degrees of restricted mobility.
2. Altered physiology and abnormal functions of most systems of the body.
3. Difficulties in resettlement in their own accommodation. Adaptations to their accommodation are invariably required and frequently re-housing is needed.
4. Loss of income due to the inability of many patients to resume work.
5. The inability of many patients to resume the same hobby and sport.
6. Uncertainty about the reactions of partners, relatives and friends.
7. Uncertainty about their sexual abilities and their ability to father their own children.
8. Uncertainty about the future.

It is fair to state that a spinal cord injury is a catastrophic event that totally disrupts an individual's life. The injury usually occurs within fractions of a second affecting the medical, physical, social and psychological state of previously normal and healthy individuals. While initially resuscitation will take priority, planning of total management care to help towards preventing and solving some or all of these problems ought to be undertaken at a very early stage by a multi-disciplinary team led by a specialist in the field in a co-ordinated, sensible and efficient manner.

The manner in which the social re-integration is conducted can be briefly described under the following headings:

### *7.1. Fact Finding About the Patient*

This starts at a very early stage, usually within the first couple of days from injury. It is a continuous process that extends over the few weeks and information is gathered from the patient, his partner, relatives and friends. The hospital team must be familiar with the patient's personal history, past history, nature of employment prior to the accident, type of accommodation, hobbies and habits, all before formulating a plan of action.

The collection of information is usually done formally by the specialist and informally by any member or members of the team over a period of 2–3 weeks. Communication between the members of the team is crucial to the process and is formally established following the weekly ward round where all the members are expected to be present.

### *7.2. Planning of Management*

The information available is assessed as to its completeness and accuracy by the whole team at Oswestry. This consists of the Specialist in charge, the Charge Nurse, the Head Physiotherapist, the Head Occupational Therapist, the Social Worker and the Coordinator. Usually by the second or third week the patient would have chosen a member of the team to whom he or she would confide. Informal counselling and support is usually given by this person as well as the Specialist in charge and the other members of the team. The patient is offered the opportunity to meet successfully rehabilitated patients with long-term paraplegia or tetraplegia, chosen and matched to him.

At an early stage, usually within the first two weeks, the patient's General Practitioner, Community Nurse, Community Physiotherapist and Occupationl Therapist, Social Worker and local Housing Department are informed by letter about the patient's condition and the assessed information. The patient is formally informed of the prognosis by the sixth week following injury. His potential abilities ought to be emphasized at least as well as his disabilities.

Resettlement in adequate accommodation is a fundamental step towards social re-integration. The discharge of a patient to accommodation unadapted for wheelchair access would result in further restriction of indoor mobility with the patient often having to live usually in one room, where sleeping, feeding, bladder emptying, bowel evacuation and entertaining of friends all occur in one place, as well as inaccessability to outdoor activities. These conditions are likely to affect the sense of dignity and the morale of a patient whose body image has already been disturbed. Not surprisingly, further depression resulting in self-neglect occurs with direct implications on the medical condition; common examples being the development of pressure sores, urinary retention and infection, contractures of joints, constipation, etc.

The resettlement process starts at about eight weeks following the injury. An experienced member of the team, usually together with the patient, visit the accommodation where a pre-arranged meeting with the local team in the patient's own area takes place. The accommodation is assessed as to its suitability for wheelchair ambulation and the required alterations or alternative re-housing highlighted. The needs of the patient and the required support are also discussed with the team of his local community. The patient must be encouraged to take an active role in these discussions. Preparations thus commence while the patient continues his rehabilitation in hospital. Frequent correspondence with the housing department and the social services is often required. The house is re-visited following adaptation or re-housing and must be passed as suitable and safe prior to discharge of the patient.

About 80% of the patients discharged from Oswestry return to their own community, either in their adapted accommodation or to a new house. The resettlement process usually results in the delay of discharge of about four to eight weeks following the completion of rehabilitation.

Problems in finding suitable accommodation occur in about 20% of patients. These either have no family or have left home and do not wish to return, but there is also an increasing number of patients with psycho-social problems prior to their accident. A half-way house is often required for these patients, usually in a Young Disabled Unit or a hospital in the area where they were living prior to their accident.

## 8. The Process of Social Re-integration

This starts while the patient is in the rehabilitative stage in hospital.

Independence in daily living activities or dependence on a caring partner are essential for a smooth, or at least minimally traumatic re-integration. Paraplegic patients are encouraged and taught by the staff to become fully independent and this is achieved in almost all cases.

It must be appreciated that the hospital environment is necessarily protective to patients who in the early stages need to meet similarly disabled persons in all stages of life. It is not surprising that initially the patients are apprehensive about leaving this environment. With good planning, however, and gentle persuasion, this feeling is overcome by the majority of the patients. Outings are organized by the staff who usually accompany groups of patients to known pubs and restaurants familiar with the physical and psychological handling of these patients. When the patient and his partner have successfully achieved a safe car transfer they are encouraged to have short trips outside the hospital on a number of occasions. At about twelve weeks following the injury, the patients are usually encouraged to use a specially adapted flat to exercise independent living with their partner or relative and gain more confidence. Once this has been successfully achieved, they are allowed home for weekends and increasing periods of time. Makeshift temporary adaptations are necessary together with communication with the local district nurse and general practitioner.

Discussion with the patient's employer is usually carried out at about three months following the injury. In our experience most employers are sympathetic and a great number of them will offer alternative employment if possible. Unfortunately, in a climate of unemployment many patients will not find employment within 18 months following the injury. A number of patients, however, have managed to develop a hobby into a gainful part time employment.

At an early stage following mobilization the patient is encouraged to take up his old hobby and sport if possible. Alternatively, this is substituted with new ones which can be attended to from a wheelchair.

It is essential from an early stage that a channel of communication be established between the specialist and the patient to aim at gaining his trust and confidence which are essential for ensuring effective management in the short and the long term.

## 9. Psychological Responses

Fear for life as well as the unknown is experienced by patients, usually in the first three weeks. This is followed by depression when the patients realize that their body functions are altered and there is no improvement. The depression deepens when confronted with the prognosis. Anger and denial usually follow only to be interrupted by episodes of reactive depression. Following a period of "bargaining" some degree of acceptance of the disability is usual. Patients with incomplete and recovering lesions usually have more difficulty in accepting their disability. These reactions are encountered in the majority of the patients with no history of psychological disturbances prior to their accident. We consider them as normal responses to a severe trauma of this nature and they require sympathy, time to listen and support by the treating clinician. In most cases, the "work" of psychological re-orientation is achieved by the "patient community".

## 10. Psychosexual Responses

### *10.1. Male Sexuality*

It must be emphasized that all young paraplegic and tetraplegic patients become apprehensive at different stages about their ability to perform sexually and their ability to father their own children. Some are more articulate than others and it is the clinician's duty to lead the shy patient to voice his apprehensions. Informal counselling is undertaken at the patient's request, usually within the first six to eight weeks following the injury. Formal counselling of the male patient and his partner is usually undertaken prior to his first weekend at home and when family planning becomes important, usually a few months to a few years following discharge.

#### Sexual Aspects of Male Patients

In general terms the libido of the paraplegic or tetraplegic patient is not diminished. It might be depressed, however, during the acute stage following the injury, mainly due to fear and apprehension. It tends to be enhanced at later stages, dreams with erotic and orgasmic contents being quite common. During the rehabilitation period, preoccupation with inadequate sexual functions and fertility are common.

Genital sensation is absent in all patients with a complete paraplegia. The patient with incomplete spinal cord injury may experience pleasant or unpleasant genital sensation during the sexual act. Patients with complete upper motor neurone lesions are able to obtain reflex erections and in general the higher the lesion the stronger and more sustained the erections are. Failure of external ejaculation occurs in the majority of patients with complete spinal cord injury and retrograde ejaculation occurs in a number of patients. However, the true incidence of this is unknown.

In our experience, sexual counselling of the patient needs to be tailored to the individual taking into account age, social up-bringing, family background, previous sexual habits, professional status and level and type of injury. Counselling is undertaken on an individual basis as well as in groups. Group counselling is valuable for the basic description of the physiological aspects and the influence of the nervous system on sexuality and fertility. Repeated individual counselling sessions at different stages during the rehabilitation programme including pre and post weekend leave from the ward are essential.

Fertility counselling is best done on an individual basis in the presence of the patient's partner. Patients with upper motor neurone lesions below the level of D 5 may use a vibrator applied at the ventral surface of the glans penis for three minutes on, three minutes off, up to forty-five minute sessions. Ejaculation occurs in about 50% of the cases. When ejaculation on demand has been established the patient attends the hospital as a day case coinciding with the ovulation period of his partner. A semen specimen is examined and the partner inseminated. Electro-ejaculation is attempted when vibro-ejaculation fails (Brindley 1984).

### *10.2. Sexual Aspects of Female Patients*

Following the onset of traumatic paraplegia, there is often a prolonged period of amenorrhea which may last for up to a year. Fertility is usually restored at the end of this period, indeed some patients have become pregnant without having had a menstrual period following their injury. The authors have inadequate experience of evaluating the significant sexual problems of female patients, Griffith and Trieschmann (1975) give a useful account.

## 11. Follow-up and Long-term Support

Following discharge from hospital the regular and frequent follow up of these patients is necessary to avoid preventable complications and to ensure the early diagnosis and management of inevitable complications. It must be appreciated that these patients have loss of sensation below the level of their lesions and their symptomatology can be misleading to the clinician who is unfamiliar with the diagnostic problems of these patients. We usually see the patient three times in the first year following discharge, twice in the second year, then every one, two or three years for the rest of their lives. A complete assessment of all systems in the body, together with a psychological and social evaluation are undertaken, usually on an outpatient basis. Problems are identified and managed vigorously (Bedbrook 1985).

## 12. Post-traumatic Syringomyelia

Although the association with spinal trauma and syringomyelia was already known, it was Barnett *et al.* (1966) who firmly established traumatic paraplegia as being a common cause of syringomyelia. Since that time Barnett and Jousse (1976), Vernon *et al.* (1982) and Rossier *et al.* (1985), together with many other authors, have given a clearer picture of the symptomatology incidence and treatment of the condition. With the introduction of newer diagnostic methods this picture is still changing.

### *12.1. Symptoms and Physical Signs*

Vernon *et al.* (1982) and Rossier *et al.* (1985) list the major symptoms as pain, sensory impairment and increasing weakness as the major presenting symptoms. Of these, pain is the presenting symptoms in well over half the cases eventually diagnosed. Vernon *et al.* (1982) report that the pain was often localized centrally over the lower cervical or upper thoracic spinous processes. It radiated into the arm or trunk. Pain was often a dull ache, it was also precipitated by coughing in many patients. Occasionally the pain was of a stabbing or burning nature.

Sensory disturbance usually consists of loss of pain and temperature sensation above the original spinal cord lesion. Rossier *et al.* (1985) and Vernon *et al.* (1982) found that it occurred at some stage in almost all the patients with post-traumatic syringomyelia. Some patients were unaware of their sensory loss until this was pointed out to them by the examining doctor. Although initially often unilateral, it was common for the condition to become bilateral and to spread to further areas. It often involved the face and this was sometimes the earliest manifestation of the condition.

Vernon *et al.* (1982) reported that eventually 70% of their cases developed some fresh motor weakness, 47.5% had unilateral upper limb weakness and 15% had bilateral upper limb weakness. The severity of the condition was variable but 2 of their patients became totally helpless as a result of their additional paralysis. Rossier *et al.* (1985) reported increased motor deficits in 40% of their patients.

Other symptoms such as increased sweating, increased spasticity and autonomic dysreflexia are also reported as sequelae of post-traumatic syringomyelia. Brain stem involvement may give rise to cranial nerve signs, hiccups and dysphagia.

### *12.2. Incidence*

This was originally considered a rare condition and Barnett *et al.* (1976) reported 2.3% amongst their paraplegic patients and 0.3% amongst their tetraplegic patients. In their retrospective study they found a higher prevalence in incomplete paraplegics than in complete paraplegics. Vernon *et al.* (1982) suggested that their reported 1.6% was an under estimate. Rossier *et al.* (1985) reported an overall incidence in his patients of 3.2% and he found 4.5% amongst his tetraplegic patients and 1.7% amongst his paraplegic patients, it seems likely that they were investigating a group of tetraplegic patients in a manner that had not previously been done by the other authors.

The onset of the initial symptoms of post-traumatic syringomyelia has been described as early as three months after the original injury and as late as 34 years.

### *12.3. Diagnosis*

Until very recently the standard method of diagnosis has been by metrizamide myelography followed by delayed CT scan. The initial myelography often reveals expansion of the cord and the delayed CT scan shows the syrinx itself. More recently magnetic resonance imaging has opened up the possibility of a non-invasive investigation of this condition. With the increasing high resolution by this technique, it should be possible to detect the majority of cases at an early stage. Gebarski *et al.* (1985) conclude that magnetic resonance imaging is the most accurative pre-operative method for detecting the condition and they recommended that this should be combined with intra-operative ultra-sonography for detecting septations and small additional cysts. Intra-operative ultra-sonography was also helpful in myelotomy positioning, shunt placement and verification of cyst decompression.

### *12.4. Progression and Treatment*

Progression of the condition is irregular and uncertain and it can remain dormant for many years after initial onset. Rossier *et al.* (1985) report 19 patients that were treated conservatively and 13 of these showed either new symptoms or a progression of their deficit over the years. Vernon *et al.* (1982) stated that "untreated, all the cases have progressed either slowly or rapidly, some to severe disability. At least 3 had brain stem involvement. 2 progressed to a quadriplegic helplessness".

### *12.5. Surgical Treatment*

Vernon *et al.* (1983) report 27 cases who had had various operations to drain the cyst. These operations were cord transection (in cases with complete spinal cord lesions), tube syringoscopy into the subarachnoid space and syringo-peritoneal shunt. Taking the results together, pain was improved in 14 patients, motor power was improved in 14 patients and there was sensory improvement in 8 patients.

Suzuki *et al.* (1985) report 17 cases of post-traumatic syringomyelia treated by syringo-peritoneal shunt. Post-operatively 14 were improved, 3 were unchanged and none were made worse.

It is apparent that the results of conservative treatment are unsatisfactory, the long term results of surgical treatment have not yet been evaluated. There is no doubt that with increasing use of magnetic resonance imaging, a substantial number of cysts will be detected and it will be reasonable to drain those producing significant symptoms or signs.

## 13. Life Expectancy

Since the 2nd World War there has been a great improvement in the life expectancy of paraplegics. The most reliable statistics come from Canada (Geisler *et al.* 1983). There figures indicate that in complete paraplegics the annual mortality is three times that of the general population. The series of papers on life expectancy from Canada show that life expectancy has improved throughout each decade, therefore, further improvement in life expectancy can be anticipated.

## 14. Conclusions

As yet there is no cure for traumatic paraplegia. Medical and surgical management of the spinal cord lesion itself can do little, if anything, to influence the outcome. In spite of this there has been an immense improvement in the management and rehabilitation of patients suffering from traumatic paraplegia since the 2nd World War. These improvements are not only in initial survival and avoidance of complications but also in respect of physical and psychological rehabilitation, transport, social re-integration and employment. These improvements have been associated with the development of specialized spinal injuries centres (Guttmann 1976) and the authors of this chapter recommend that a patient with a spinal cord injury should be admitted to such a centre at the earliest possible moment and unless there is a full neurological recovery, he should remain under the supervision of that centre for the rest of his life.

## References

1. Barnett HJM, Bottrell EH, Jousse AT, Wynne Jones M (1966) Progressive myelopathy as a sequel of traumatic paraplegia. Brain 89: 159–174
2. Barnett HJM, Jousse AT (1976) Posttraumatic syringomyelia (cystic myelopathy). In: Vinken PJ, Bruyn GW (eds) Handbook of Clinical Neurology, vol 26. North Holland, Amsterdam, pp 113–157
3. Bedbrook G (ed) (1985) Lifetime care of the paraplegic patient. Churchill Livingstone, Edinburgh
4. Bohlman HH (1979) Acute fractures and dislocations of the cervical spine. J Bone Joint Surg 61a: 1119–1142

5. Bohlman HH, Freehafer A, Dejak J (1985) The results of treatment of acute injuries of the upper thoracic spine with paralysis. J Bone Joint Surg 67a: 360 – 369
6. Bracken MB, Webb SB, Wagner FC (1978) Classification of the severity of acute spinal cord injury: Implications for management. Paraplegia 15: 319 – 326
7. Brindley GS (1984) The fertility of men with spinal injuries. Paraplegia 22: 337 – 348
8. Bromley I (1985) Tetraplegia and paraplegia: a guide for physiotherapists. 3rd ed. Churchill Livingstone, Edinburgh
9. Burke DC, Burley HT, Ungar GH (1985) Data of spinal injuries—part II. Outcome of the treatment of 352 consecutive admissions. Aust NZ J Surg 55: 377 – 382
10. Cardozo L, Krishnan KR, Polkey CE, Rushton DN, Brindley GS (1984) Urodynamic observations on patients with sacral anterior root stimulators. Paraplegia 22: 201 – 209
11. Chehrazi B, Wagner FC, Collins WF, Freeman DH (1981) A scale for evaluation of spinal cord injury. J Neurosurg 54: 310 – 315
12. El Masri WS, Silver JR (1981) Prophylactic anticoagulant therapy in patients with spinal cord injury. Paraplegia 19: 334 – 342
13. Frankel HL (1967) Bowel training. Paraplegia 4: 254 – 256
14. Frankel HL (1969) Ascending cord lesion in the early stages following spinal injury. Paraplegia 7: 111 – 118
15. Frankel HL, Hancock DO, Hyslop G, Melzak J, Michaelis LS, Ungar GH, Vernon JDS, Walsh JJ (1969) The value of postural reduction in the initial management of closed injuries of the spine with paraplegia and tetraplegia. Paraplegia 7: 179 – 192
16. Frankel HL, Michaelis LS, Golding DR, Beral V (1972) The Blood pressure in paraplegia. Paraplegia 10: 193 – 198
17. Frankel HL, Mathias CJ (1976) The cardiovascular system in tetraplegia and paraplegia. In: Vinken PJ, Bruyn GW (eds) Handbook of Clinical Neurology, vol 26. North Holland, Amsterdam, pp 313 – 333
18. Frankel HL, Mathias CJ (1979) Cardiovascular aspects of autonomic dysreflexia since Guttmann and Whitteridge (1947). Paraplegia 17: 46 – 51
19. Gebarski SS, Maynard FW, Gabrielsen TO, Knake JE, Latack JT, Hoff JT (1985) Post-traumatic progressive myelopathy. Radiology 157: 379 – 385
20. Geisler WO, Jousse AT, Wynne-Jones M, Breithaupt D (1983) Survival in traumatic spinal cord injury. Paraplegia 21: 364 – 373
21. Griffith ER, Trieschmann RB (1975) Sexual functioning in women with spinal cord injury. Arch Phys Med Rehabil 56: 18 – 21
22. Guttmann L (1976) Spinal cord injuries: Comprehensive management and research. 2nd ed. Blackwell, Oxford
23. Mathias CJ, Frankel HL (1983) Autonomic failure in tetraplegia. In: Bannister R (ed) Autonomic failure: a textbook of clinical disorders of the autonomic nervous system OUP, pp 453 – 488
24. Perkash I (1978) Experience with the management of thrombo-embolism with spinal cord injuries. Part I. Incidence, diagnosis and role of some risk factors. Paraplegia 16: 322 – 331

25. Rossier AB, Foo D, Shillito J, Dyro FM (1985) Post-traumatic cervical syringomyelia. Brain 108: 439–461
26. Suzuki M, Davis C, Symon L, Gentile F (1985) Syringo-peritoneal shunt for treatment of cord cavitation. J Neurol Neurosurg Psychiatry 48: 620–627
27. Vernon JB, Silver JR, Ohry A (1982) Post-traumatic syringomyelia. Paraplegia 20: 339–364
28. Vernon JD, Silver JR, Symon L (1983) Post-traumatic syringomyelia: The results of surgery. Paraplegia 21: 37–46
29. Walsh JJ, Tribe LR (1965) Phlebothrombosis and pulmonary embolism in paraplegia. Paraplegia 3: 209–213
30. Watson N (1978) Anticoagulant therapy in the prevention of venous thrombosis and pulmonary embolism in the spinal cord injury. Paraplegia 16: 265–269
31. Wilmot CB, Hall K (1986) Evaluation of acute surgical intervention in traumatic paraplegia. Paraplegia 24: 71–76
32. Young JS, Dexter WR (1978) Neurological recovery distal to the zone of injury in 172 cases of closed, traumatic spinal cord injury. Paraplegia 16: 39–49

# Revascularisation of the Traumatised Spinal Cord: Experimental and Clinical

J. Abraham

C.M.C. Hospital, Vellore (India)

## Contents



## 1. Introduction

Since the time of the Edwin Smith Papyrus (ca. 1700 B.C.), paraplegia has been considered one of the most depressing clinical states to manage and has consequently been a challenge to the basic research worker and the clinician (Collins 1983, Harris 1985).

Interest was kindled by early investigators like Spiller (1899); and in the last fifteen years, probably related to a global increase in the problem, there has been a veritable explosion in our knowledge of spinal cord injuries.

Progress has been impeded by deficiencies in the appreciation of the basic biochemical and cellular phenomena associated with central nervous system trauma and a sense of unfounded hopelessness in regard to the plasticity and regenerative capabilities of the traumatised spinal cord, unwittingly reinforced by the superb rehabilitation of such patients, pioneered by Sir Ludwig Guttmann, Howard Rusk, and Sir George

Bedbrook. However, in the last decade, public opinion, governments and in particular private agencies have provided the necessary impetus for a resurgence in interest for a more critical and scientific look at cellular events combined with a more positive approach to therapy.

In our understanding of spinal cord trauma in patients we felt that both contusion and compression play an equally important role in the initial and subsequent pathophysiology of neuronal and vascular changes. The subsequent discussion emphasises the management of the injured spinal cord by means of a pedicled omental onlay graft, as one possible mode of treatment for acute and chronic spinal cord injured patients.

## 2. Experimental Studies

There are two major types of models of spinal cord injury currently being utilised in laboratories; modifications of the Allen model (1911, 1914), which essentially causes an acute contusion injury by a weight dropped from a specific height onto a laminectomised segment of dura covered spinal cord and a compressive injury model employing an extradural balloon as described by Tarlov (1953) or a circumferential sleeve compression and a spring clip, Deecke and Tator (1973), Rivlin and Tator (1978). In our laboratory we have been able to produce a fairly reproducible primate model of contusion by the Allen technique, utilising a 20 gm weight drop from a height of 20 cms and a model of compression produced by placing a 20 gm weight on the spinal cord (Abraham 1985).

If the Oslerian truism "as is our pathology so our practise" was given heed to by workers in the field of spinal cord injury, perhaps a more logical combination of therapy would have evolved. The pathological changes related to the mechanics of the force generated and applied to the spinal cord at the moment of injury resulting in physical alteration of neuronal, axonal and vascular integrity in the first few minutes to hours are considered to be primary pathological changes. These primary changes merge with a cascade of inter-related events which are physical and biochemical in nature and constitute the all important secondary changes. The physical changes are alteration in blood perfusion, oedema formation, increase in tissue pressure, and a drop in pH resulting from a local increase in the concentration of lactic acid and carbon dioxide. The biochemical changes are primarily related to dislocation and imbalance of neurotransmitters, abnormalities of the cell membrane with $Na^+$, $K^+$, ATPase changes, lysosomal enzyme activation and release, intracellular influx of $Ca^{++}$ and initiation of free radical pathology. Remote effects on adjacent supposedly normal nontraumatised spinal cord have also been noted by us.

Pathophysiological changes in respect of some physical and biochemical parameters in a primate spinal cord contusion model compared to sham operated controls in our laboratories showed a significant increase of water content up to 48 hours at which time the experiment was terminated. The percentage increase in water was greater during the first 4 hours of injury compared to the period from 24–48 hours (Theodore *et al.* 1984, 1985).

Lipid peroxidation assessed by measuring malonaldehyde by the thiobarbituric method showed a significant increase up to 2 hours, then at 8, 24, and 48 hours and not at other time periods Abraham *et al.* (1985). Histamine, on the other hand, showed a significant elevation up to 4 hours and a decrease from 8 hours to 24 hours. Norepinephrine levels were minimally elevated up to 4 hours and significantly so at 8 hours after which no increase was detected up to 48 hours (Kurvilla *et al.* 1985). The following lysosomal enzymes β D. Hexosaminidase, α-L-fucosidase, α-D-Mannosidase and β-D-galactosidase showed an elevation at all time periods studied (Abraham *et al.* 1985). The most important factor which emerges from these studies is that each of the parameters seem to be time-bound and if appropriate therapy is to be instituted careful attention to time after trauma is imperative.

The late pathological sequelae are degeneration, repair, scar formation, traumatic axonal swelling, syringomyelic cavities and arachnoiditis, with or without narrowing of the bony spinal canal, and is probably the most neglected area of SCI pathology.

## 3. Treatment of Spinal Cord Injury Patients

### *3.1. Principles*

Both the physical injury and the secondary pathologic sequelae are equally important factors and attention to one with exclusion of the other or attention directed only to spinal stabilisation with no consideration of the intrinsic pathology of the cord has unfortunately been a common practice in the management of SCI patients. Until the present time the treatment of SCI patients has usually not taken into account the combined management of the acute, intermediate and late sequelae of spinal cord injury. On theoretical considerations it would seem that treatment in the acute phases of spinal cord trauma should comprise measures directed towards the control of local haemorrhagic necrosis of grey matter, local oedema and neutralisation of secondary changes; and treatment of the chronic stage should emphasise revascularisation of the spinal cord and prevention of arachnoiditis. Though no definite therapeutic measure is available which could achieve the above ideal, preliminary data from this laboratory and from patients are accumulating which suggest that myelotomy with omental transposition in the acute stage and myelolysis with omental transposition may provide the essential requirements in the management of the acute and chronic spinal cord injuries respectively.

### 3.2. Spinal Cord Revascularisation

The rationale for spinal cord revascularisation is based on the general acceptance of the fact that following trauma there is early and late ischaemia at the site of injury Bingham (1975), Crawford (1977), Dohrmann (1975), Ducker (1976, 1971, 1978), Griffiths (1976), Kobrine (1975), Sandler (1976), Smith (1978). Rupture of intrinsic grey matter capillaries occurs followed by immediate extravasation of blood, reduction of capillary blood flow and changes in white matter blood flow. Some areas in the white matter may show a decrease in blood flow, while other areas may have an increase in blood flow. In perfusion studies conducted on SCI primates in our laboratory (unpublished data) we have shown not only a marked reduction of capillary perfusion at the site of injury but also in adjacent non-traumatised segments at a distance of 1–2 cms from the contused area. In acute spinal cord trauma vascular perfusion of the spinal cord may be reduced by systemic hypotension from surgical shock. We believe that the major factor in the rupture of intrinsic grey matter capillaries is the physical impact force resulting in a mechanical deformation stress too great for the blood vessels to sustain. The subsequent changes both in the grey and white matter following the initial insult are secondary and dependent on local vasoactive substances, reaction of the vascular intima, platelet aggregability and vasogenic oedema. The result of the intrinsic blood vessel damage resulting in haemorrhage and oedema, is a rapid build up of tissue pressure within the cord which secondarily causes further ischaemia. Such a hypothesis proposed more than 40 years ago by Freeman and Wright (1953) and by Joyness and Freeman (1963) when tried on experimental animals demonstrated improvement following myelotomy and the use of hypertonic solutions.

It is generally accepted that ischaemia and oedema may be the two most important factors in the initiation of secondary injury (Griffiths 1976, Wagner 1978, Stewart and Wagner 1979); the latter group have demonstrated spread of post-traumatic oedema along the white matter tracts over a few segments. In studies conducted in our laboratories on a primate contusion (20 gm × 20 cms) injury model the water content estimated by the wet-weight-dry weight method showed an increase up to 48 hours when the experiment was terminated. On the other hand a 20 gm compression even for a period of 8 hours did not cause an increase in water content, whereas decompression caused a significant increase in water content. The development of oedema is a manifestation of an increased permeability of the blood brain barrier. The increase in blood brain barrier permeability following contusion injury and decompression following compression is caused by many factors including increase in local concentrations of amines like histamine (Kuruvilla and Abraham 1985) which increase permeability of blood vessels. A pedicled omental onlay graft onto the traumatised spinal cord immediately following injury was done in our laboratory, and a comparison of the water content between treated and untreated monkeys, showed a statistically significant reduction in the water content of the spinal cord in the group with the omental graft. The ability of the omentum to absorb fluid, has been utilised to drain hydrocephalus via lumbo-omental shunts using the vascular omental pedicle, Wennerstrand (1974), Levander (1978).

We are unable to state categorically that reduction in oedema alone helps in reversing or reducing the quantum of neurological damage and is of significance in preserving neurological function, though one could assume that such is the case.

The ability of the pedicled omentum to revascularise normal and traumatised spinal cords has been reported by Goldsmith *et al.* (1975, 1983). He clearly demonstrated in dogs and cats vascular connections between the omentum and the pia-arachnoid and via these connections into the intrinsic blood vessels of the cord.

In our laboratories we have been able to confirm that pedicled omental transposition onto the primate spinal cord achieves absorption of oedema from the contused area of the spinal cord and provides an added means of vascular supply to the cord (Theodore *et al.* 1984).

Special properties of capillary ingrowth by the omentum has been investigated in animals and a firm adhesion was demonstrated between the omentum and underlying tissue occuring between 14 and 24 hours and capillary ingrowth in 3 or 4 days; confirmed by Thompson (1945), Myllasniemi (1968) and Eliska (1968). In order to form an effective collateral circulation in coronary occlusion Beck and Tychy (1935) and O'Shaugnessy (1937) developed pericardial adhesions in dogs with the aid of the omentum. O'Shaugnessy in 1937 and Hunter in 1938 performed omento-cardiopexy with limited success in patients with cardiac insufficiency. The interested reader may refer to the book, entitled "The Greater Omentum" edited by D. Liebermann-Meffert and Harvey White, Springer-Verlag 1983, for an update review of the properties of the omentum and its surgical application in the experimental and clinical situation.

Goldsmith (1985) found that placement of the intact omentum upon a recently traumatised spinal cord was effective in lessening motor and neuroelectrical dysfunction in a group of cats.

One of the features of the late sequelae of spinal cord injury is the symptoms of progressive myelopathy, described by Barnett *et al.* (1966), Wozniewicz (1977), Shannon *et al.* (1981) and Vernon (1982). Experimental models of spinal cord injury also showed essentially the same features, Balentine (1978), Kao *et al.* (1977), Kao *et al.* (1977). Essentially there is arachnoiditis which may be localised or may involve a long segment and syringomyelic cavitation of the spinal cord with varying degrees of loss of neuronal tissue, gliosis and scar formation. The pattern of traumatic necrosis which results in post-traumatic syringomyelia is probably the result of intraspinal vascular injury, and data on human autopsy material supports this view.

Perovitch (1983) examined 125 chronic paraplegics both radiologically and at operation or autopsy and detected cavitations, atrophy, adhesions and vascular alterations as the main pathological changes. In the few cases of chronic paraplegia which we have observed at surgery, ischaemia of the spinal cord appeared to be very likely, occurring as a result of arachnoidal adhesions or secondary to syringomyelic cavitation. The surgical management of syringomyelia as summarised by Vernon *et al.* (1983) was cord transection in complete paraplegia and tube syringotomy either to the subarachnoid space or to the peritoneal cavity.

### *3.3. Omental Transposition*

Omental transposition to the injured spinal cord in patients has been done at C.M.C. hospital, Vellore since 1982. It was performed on four patients with acute injuries and on 7 chronic paraplegic patients.

The *indications* for omental transposition have been as follows:

1. All acute fracture dislocation of the thoraco-lumbar spine with complete paraplegia, seen within 6–8 hours of injury.

2. Chronic traumatic paraplegia with minimal motor or sensory preservation, *e.g.*, just movement of a toe; associated with an almost complete block on myelography.

*Pre-operative preparation:* Informed consent is obtained from the patient and relatives and routine preparation for spinal and abdominal surgery is made, with special attention to bladder and bowel functions, and to the patient's respiratory state.

*Operative procedure:* Under general anaesthesia, the patient is placed in the left lateral position with his back 90° to the floor, and secured to the operating table in such a way as to allow a 10–15° tilt of the right shoulder forwards or back as required. Two teams of surgeons may work simultaneously at the abdominal and spinal sites. In patients with acute traumatic paraplegia, spinal cord decompression is done first, whereas in chronic paraplegia, the abdomen is opened first and the omentum mobilised.

*Mobilising the omentum:* The omentum is lifted up to open the lesser sac through the posterior part of the greater omentum. The plane of dissection is usually on the caudal mesenteric border of the transverse colon where it is avascular and easy to separate. Sharp dissection is used and haemostasis is important. After the attachment of the omentum has been separated from the transverse colon the separation from the greater curvature of the stomach from left to right is undertaken leaving it pedicled to the right gastro epiploic artery. The gastro—epiploic arcade is incorporated in the mobilised omentum utilising the technique described by Alday and Goldsmith (1972). The omentum is lengthened by cutting between the vascular arcades preserving the blood supply to the distal end (Das 1976) and brought subcutaneously to the spinal cord site, facilitated by one or two incisions between the abdominal and spinal incisions. The spinal cord exposure is made by a downward "C" shaped incision, the dome of the "C" being about 2–3 inches from the midline and the two ends of "C" 2–3 vertebra above and below the region of the block. The incision on the back is deepened down to the muscle layer and the skin and subcutaneous tissue flap are reflected to expose the midline and the paraspinal muscle. A subperiosteal reflection of the paraspinal muscles is done and they are held aside by self-retaining retractors. The appropriate laminectomy is done, and the dura is opened and excised. The operating microscope is now utilised to facilitate dissection of the arachnoid. A paramedian myelotomy is made in acute cases and also in chronic cases when a traumatic syringomyelic cavity is diagnosed. The omentum is now placed on to the surface of the spinal cord and held in place by sutures taken through the cut end of the dura and the omentum. The abdominal and back incisions are closed in the usual fashion without a drain.

### *3.4. Summary of Clinical Details of Operated Patients*

All four acute cases were completely paralysed with motor, sensory and autonomic loss and the injured segments were between $D_{10}$ and $L_1$.

The seven chronic paraplegics had varying degrees of motor, sensory and autonomic preservation with differing patterns of contracture, disuse atrophy of muscles and were all confined to wheel chairs. The length of time after the accident varied from 3 months to 3 years (approximately). All had complete or near complete block on myelography due to arachnoiditis with or without cystic changes in the cord.

On follow up for two years after surgery, two out of four acute paraplegics were able to walk, one without any support and the other with below knee calipers and crutches. Five out of seven chronic paraplegics had improved in their muscle strength by about two grades and were able to walk with calipers and crutches.

## 4. Conclusions

In our attempts at revascularisation of the traumatised spinal cord by a pedicled omental onlay graft we felt that the omentum would not only provide new vascular channels to the pial surface but also prevent recurrence of arachnoidal adhesions and facilitate CSF absorption from the syringomyelic cavities once they were surgically opened. We felt that the latter use of the omentum would perhaps be superior to the current technique of syringostomies. Our preliminary results with the use of the omental graft in the management of syringomyelia of non-traumatic origin (4 cases) also supports the use in the post-traumatic myelopathic situation.

## References


1. Abraham J, Balasubramanian AS, Theodore DR, Nagarajan S (1985) Spinal cord oedema, 5 hydroxytryptamine, lipid peroxidation and lysosomal enzyme release after acute contusion and compression injury in primates. Central Nervous System Trauma vol 2 (1), pp 50–58
2. Alday ES, Goldsmith HS (1972) Surgical technique for omental lenthening based on arterial anatomy. Surg Gynecol Obstet 135: 103–107
3. Allen AR (1914) Remarks on the histopathological changes in the spinal cord due to impact. An experimental study. J Nerv Ment Dis 41: 141–147
4. Allen AR (1911) Surgery of experimental lession of spinal cord equivalent to crush injury of fracture dislocation of spinal column. JAMA 57: 878–890
5. Balentine JD (1978) Pathology of experimental spinal cord trauma. Laborat Invest 39: 236
6. Barnett HJM, Bottrell EH, Jouse AT, Wynn Jones M (1966) Progressive myelopathy as a sequel to traumatic paraplegia. Brain 89: 159–174
7. Beck CS, Tichy VL (1935) The production of a collateral circulation to the heart. An experimental study. Am Heart J 10: 849–873
8. Bingham WG, Goldman H, Friedman SJ, Murphy S, Yashon D, Hunt WE (1975) Blood flow in normal and injured monkey spinal cord. J Neurosurg 43: 162–171
9. Crawford RA, Griffiths IR, McCulloch J (1977) The effect of norepinephrine on the spinal cord circulation and its possible implications in the pathogenesis of acute spinal trauma. J Neurosurg 47: 567–576
10. Collins WF (1983) A review and update of experimental and clinical studies of spinal cord injury. Paraplegia 21: 204–219
11. Das SK (1976) The size of the human omentum and methods of lengthening it for transplantation. Br J Plast Surg 29: 170–174
12. Dohrmann GJ, Allen WE (1975) Microcirculation of traumatized spinal cord: a correlation of microangiography and blood flow patterns in transitory and permanent paraplegia. J Trauma 15: 1003–1013
13. Ducker TB (1976) Experimental injury of the spinal cord. In: Vinken P, Bruyn GW (eds) Handbook of clinical neurology vol 25, pp 9–26
14. Ducker TB, Perot PL (1971) Spinal cord oxygen and blood flow in trauma. Surg Forum 22: 413–415
15. Ducker TB, Solomon M, Lucas JT, Garrison WB, Perot PL (1978) Blood flow tissue oxygen, evoked potentials in both paretic and plegic monkeys. Surg Neurol 10: 64–70

16. Eliska O (1968) Blood flow in the revascularized kidney. J Cardiovasc Surg (Torino) 9: 342–347
17. Freeman LW, Wright TW (1953) Experimental observations of concussion and contusion of the spinal cord. Am Surg 137: 433–443
18. Goldsmith HS, Duckett S, Chen WF (1975) Spinal cord vascularization by intact omentum. Am J Surg 129: 262–265
19. Goldsmith HS, Steward E, Chen WF, Duckett S (1983) Application of intact omentum to the normal and traumatised spinal cord. In: Kao CC, Bunge RP, Reir RJ (eds) Spinal cord reconstruction. Raven Press, New York
20. Goldsmith HS, Steward E, Duckett S (1985) Early application of pedicled omentum to the acutely traumatised spinal cord. Paraplegia 23: 100–112
21. Griffiths IR (1976) Spinal cord blood flow after acute experimental cord injury in dogs. J Neurol Sci 27: 247–259
22. Harris P (1985) Acute spinal cord injury patients – Who cares? Paraplegia 23: 1–7
23. Hunter JB (1938–1939) Cardio-Omentupexy. Proc R Soc Med 32: 436–437
24. Joynes J, Freeman LW (1963) Urea and spinal cord trauma. Neurology 13: 69–72
25. Kao CC, Chang LW (1977) The mechanisms of spinal cord cavitation following spinal cord transection, part 1: a correlated histochemical study. J Neurosurg 46: 197
26. Kao CC, Cheng LW, Bloodworth JMB Jr (1977), part 2: electron microscopic observations. J Neurosurg 46: 745
27. Kobrine AI, Doyle TF, Martins AN (1975) Local spinal cord blood flow in experimental traumatic myelopathy. J Neurosurg 42: 144–149
28. Kuruvilla A, Theodore DR, Abraham J (1985) Norepinephrine and histamine in spinal cord trauma. Central nervous system trauma vol 2, (1), pp 69–71
29. Levander B, Asord PE (1978) Lumbo-omental shunt for drainage of cerebrospinal fluid—an experimental radionuclide study in dogs. Acta Neurochir (Wien) 43: 251–262
30. Myllarniemi H, Karppinen V (1968) Vascular pattern of peritoneal adhesions. Br J Surg 55: 605–608
31. O'Shaugnessy L (1937) Surgical treatment of cardiac ischaemia. Lancet i: 185–194
32. Perovitch M (1983) Neuroradiology of the sequelae of spinal cord trauma. Acta Neurochir (Wien) [Suppl] 32: 91–94
33. Rivlin AS, Tator CH (1978) Effect of duration of acute spinal cord compression in a new acute cord injury model in the rat. Surg Neurol 10: 39–43
34. Sandler AN, Tator CH (1976) Effect of acute spinal cord compression injury on regional spinal cord blood flow in primates. J Neurosurg 45: 660–676
35. Sandler AN, Tator CH (1976) Review of the effect of spinal cord trauma on the vessels and blood flow in the spinal cord. J Neurosurg 45: 638–646
36. Shannon N, Symon L, Logue V *et al* (1981) Clinical features, investigation and treatment of post-traumatic syringomyelia. J Neurol Neurosurg Psychiatry 44: 35–42

37. Smith AJK, McCreery DB, Bloedel JR, Chon SN (1978) Hyperemia, Co2 responsiveness, and autoregulation in the white matter following experimental spinal cord injury. J Neurosurg 48: 239 – 251
38. Spiller WG (1899) A critical summary of recent literature on concussion of the spinal cord with some original observations. Am J Med Sci 118: 190 – 198
39. Stewart WB, Wagner FC (1979) Vascular permeability changes in contused feline spinal cord. Brain Res 169: 163 – 167
40. Tator CH, Deeke L (1973) Value of normothermic perfusion, hypothermic perfusion and durotomy in the treatment of experimental acute spinal trauma. J Neurosurg 39: 52 – 64
41. Tator CH, Meguro K, Rowed DW (1982) Favorable results with syringo-subarachnoid shunts for treatment of synringomyelia. J Neurosurg 53: 517 – 523
42. Tarlov IM, Klinger H, Vitales S (1953) Spinal cord compression studies: I. experimental techniques to produce acute and gradual compression. Arch Neurol Psychiatry 70: 813 – 819
43. Theodore DR, Abraham J (1985) Indian J Med Res 81: 209 – 214
44. Theodore DR, Abraham J (1984) Possible role of transposed pedicled omentum: In the reduction of ischaemic and traumatic central nervous system oedema. In: Mohanty S, Dey PK (eds) Brain Edema Symposium Proceedings. XXXIV Annual Conference of Neurological Society of India. Dec 19 – 22, 1984 Varanasi
45. Thompson SA, Pollock B (1945) The use of the omental grafts in the thorax. An experimental study. Am J Surg 70: 227 – 231
46. Vernon JD, Silver JR, Ohry A (1982) Paraplegia 20: 339 – 364
47. Vernon JD, Silver JR, Symon L (1983) Paraplegia 21: 37 – 46
48. Wagner FC, Vangilder JC, Dohrmann GJ (1978) Pathological changes from acute to chronic in experimental spinal cord trauma. J Neurosurg 48: 92 – 98
49. Wenerstrand Jr, Levander BE (1974) Lumbo-omental drainage of cerebrospinal fluid. Acta Chir Scand 140: 91 – 94
50. Wozniewicz B (1977) Primary and secondary changes in post-traumatic myelopathy. Proceedings of International symposium on acute Management and rehabilitation after spinal cord Injuries. Konstancin, Poland, pp 15 – 27

# Sonography of Traumatic Cranial Hemorrhage

R. McLaurin[1] and Diane S. Babcock[2]

Departments of [1] Neurosurgery, [2] Radiology, and [2] Pediatrics, Children's Hospital Medical Center and the University of Cincinnati College of Medicine, Cincinnati, Ohio (U.S.A.)

With 7 Figures

## Contents



## 1. Introduction

A large body of literature has accumulated during the past decade concerning the value of sonography in the diagnosis of intracranial hemorrhage in neonates. Most of this literature has dealt with the hemorrhages of germinal matrix origin occurring in the premature infant[1-10]. There has been very little written about the value of this diagnostic modality in the management of traumatic intracranial hemorrhage. For example, in a recently published monograph on pediatric head trauma there is only one illustration of a sonogram and no description of its use as a diagnostic tool[11]. This is partially related to the relative infrequency of traumatic hemorrhage in infancy. It seems appropriate, therefore, to review the role of sonography in craniocerebral trauma of infancy.

## 2. Extracranial Hemorrhage

Extracranial hemorrhage in the newborn may occur in one of three layers. Considerable confusion has occurred regarding terminology of extracranial accumulations, but regardless of the terms applied, the location of the lesion can usually be determined clinically.

The most superficial location is in the subcutaneous tissues between the skin and the epicranial aponeurosis. This has been classically referred to as caput succedaneum and is considered to be the result of circulatory stasis in the scalp secondary to direct pressure or to the pressure difference between the intrauterine and extrauterine compartments during presentation and the birth process. The most frequent location is at the vertex of the head.

The next deeper layer in which hemorrhage may occur is between the galea and the pericranium. Since this is a continuous space over the entire scalp, blood may spread in this layer extensively. It is limited only by the attachment of the galea to the frontalis and the occipital muscles and laterally at the zygomatic arch and the auricular muscles. Considerable blood volume may be lost in the neonate into this space.

The innermost extracranial layer is between the pericranium and the skull. The pericranium is, of course, attached at the bone margins and, therefore, blood does not spread beyond the suture lines in this compartment. It is most likely to occur over the parietal bones.

On sonography, extracranial hemorrhage is seen as a mildly echogenic mass separating the scalp from the bony skull (Fig. 1). When scanning is performed over the site of the hematoma, reverberation lines parallelling the skull can be seen within the calvarium and should not be mistaken for a subdural hematoma. With artifactual reverberations, there is no shift of the midline echoes as should be seen with an intracranial mass. When the patient is scanned from the side opposite to the hematoma, the reverberation lines are seen outside of the head. A caput succedaneum or subgaleal hematoma can be differentiated from a cephalohematoma by the extension of the hematoma across the suture line.

Extracranial hemorrhage or edema of the scalp, particularly if it occurs

---

Fig. 1. Cephalohematoma. Three day old infant with swelling over right parietal region noted at birth. A) Axial scan shows cephalohematoma (*CH*) in right posterior parietal region with separation of scalp (open arrow) from bony skull (*B*) by hematoma. Reverberation lines (*R*) parallelling skull, apparently within calvarium are thought to be artifactual, but are suspicious for subdural hematoma although there is no shift of midline echoes. B) Axial scan from opposite side shows reverberation lines outside of head. (Reproduced with permission from: Babcock DS, Han BK, and LeQuesne GW, AJR 134: 457–461, 1980)

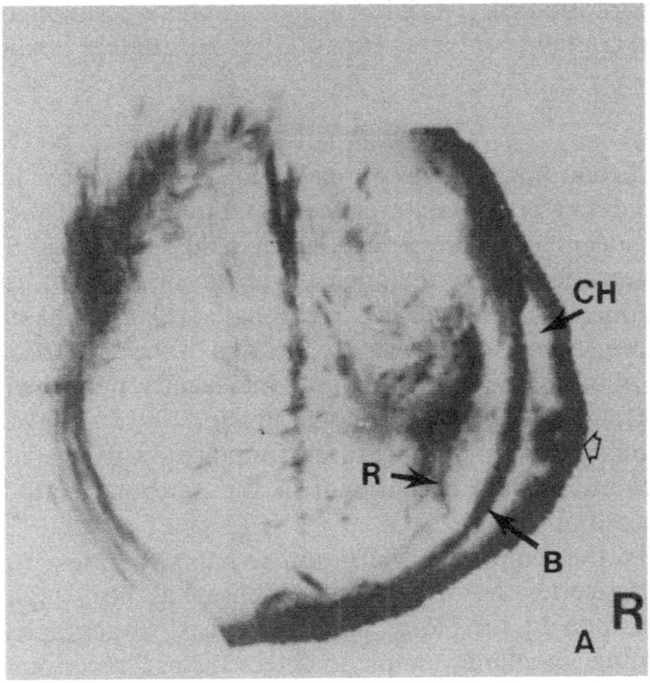


Fig. 1 A

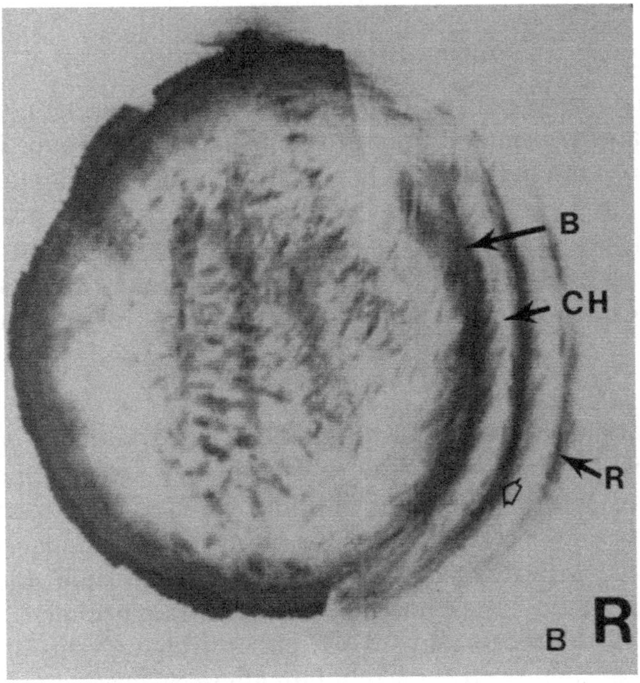


Fig. 1 B

over the anterior fontanelle, can cause significant reverberation artifacts so that the intracranial contents cannot be adequately evaluated by sonography.

## 3. Extradural Hemorrhage

Extradural hematomas are exceptionally rare in the newborn infant. The reason for this rarity is probably related to the tendency of the newborn skull to bend under external pressure rather than the splintering effect which may lead to laceration of the meningeal arteries. In addition, the dura is rather firmly adherent at the site of the coronal and lambdoid sutures and there is, therefore, less opportunity for separation of the dura from the inner skull table to allow blood accumulation. In recently published series of epidural hematomas in the pediatric age group, 10–15% have occurred below the age of 2 years and they are rarely found below the age of 1 year[3, 7]. Extradural hematomas are exceptional in the newborn period and are usually discovered at autopsy.

As in adults, the temporal localization remains the most frequent in infants. In some series, however, the incidence has been higher in the parietal region than in the lower temporal areas. Sonography has the limitation of being sometimes unable to detect surface hematomas high in the parietal area, although temporal fossa hematomas can easily be detected by this means.

## 4. Subdural Hemorrhage

Subdural hematoma is probably the most frequently occurring intracranial hematoma of *traumatic* origin in the pediatric age group. It may occur in the newborn infant as a result of birth trauma or later in infancy. It is widely held at the present time that the subdural hematoma occurring after the newborn period is most frequently a consequence of infant abuse. Early diagnosis and treatment of subdural hematomas may avoid significant damage to the underlying brain resulting in psychomotor impairment[8].

### *4.1. Acute*

While subdural hematomas may originate from arterial or venous bleeding, it is probable that those occurring in infancy are principally of venous origin. Two sources of venous bleeding are identified: tearing of bridging veins between the cerebrum and the dural sinuses, and laceration of sinuses associated with tearing of the falx and/or tentorium. Bleeding from dural sinuses may occur supratentorially or infratentorially[2]. While the trauma of the birth process may involve either bridging veins or dural sinuses, it seems likely that the trauma of infant abuse, such as occurs in the shaken baby syndrome, is most likely to affect the bridging veins.

The occurrence of subdural hematomas in the neonatal period after birth

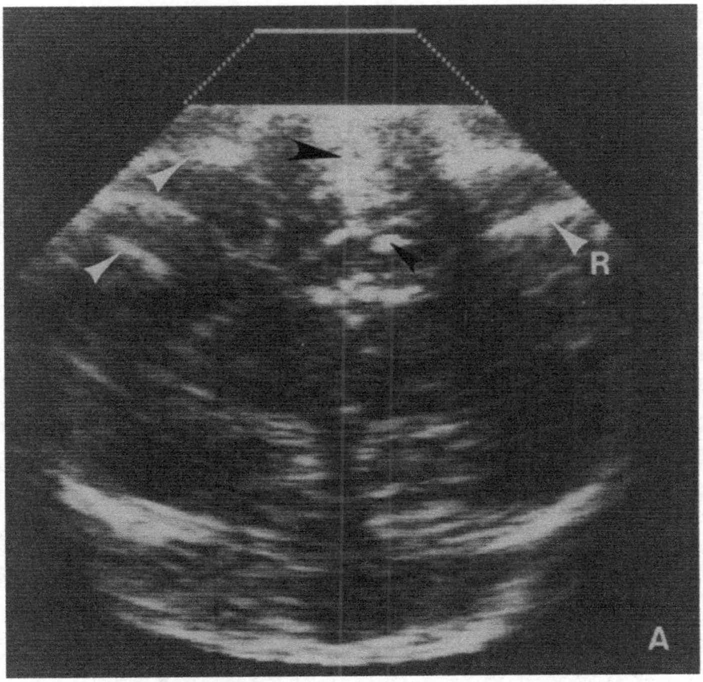


Fig. 2 A

Fig. 2. Acute subdural and subarachnoid hemorrhage. Five month old victim of child abuse. A) Coronal sonogram shows widening and increased echogenicity of interhemispheric fissure and sulci (black arrowheads) due to blood in subdural and subarachnoid spaces. Linear echogenic reverberation artifacts (white arrowheads) due to extensive scalp edema and subgaleal hematoma. B) Magnified view using 7.5 MHz transducer shows more clearly echogenic blood in the interhemispheric fissure and extraaxial spaces (arrowheads) compared to relatively hypoechoic gyri (*G*). C) and D) Higher cuts from CT scan on same day show subdural, subarachnoid, and subgaleal hematomas

trauma has been documented and defined relatively recently. The incidence is increased by difficult delivery and by breech delivery and occurs more commonly in primipara than in multipara. Molding of the skull, particularly in the occipital region, may cause laceration of the junction of the tentorium with the falx or the junction with the convexity dura. Since these junctions are the sites of major dural sinuses, subdural hematomas may ensue. It is the result of this mechanism that leads to the occurrence of subtentorial subdural hematomas in the neonatal period[2].

Clinically, the symptom of subdural bleeding from birth trauma is usually noted within the first 24 hours. Blood loss intracranially results in pallor and anemia. Compression of the cerebrum or brain stem by the hematoma may lead to seizures, extraocular deviation, hemiparesis, and

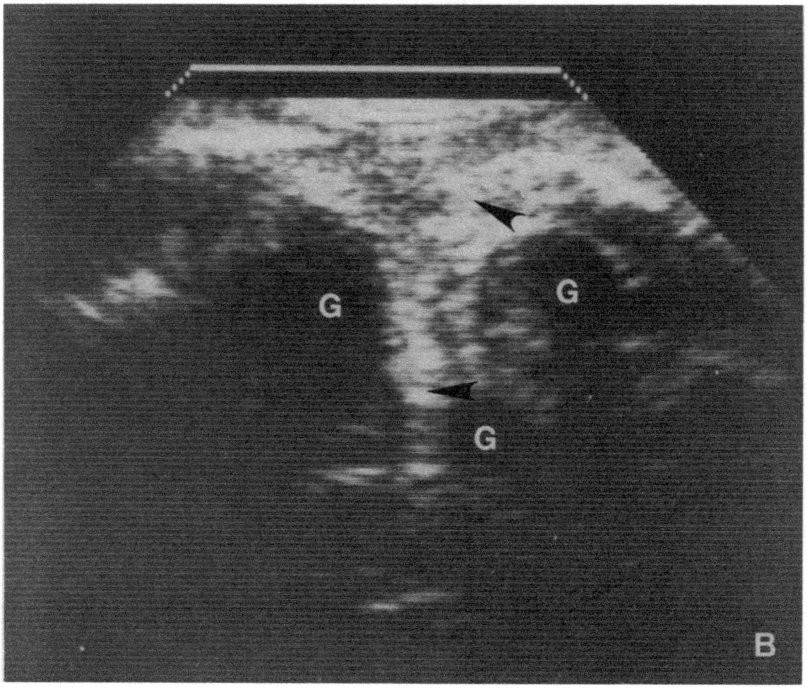


Fig. 2 B

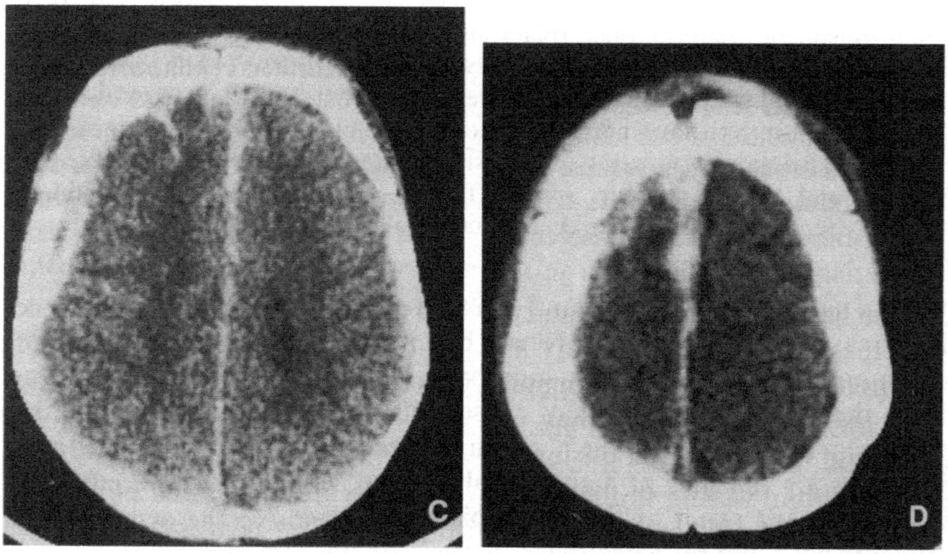


Fig. 2 C–D

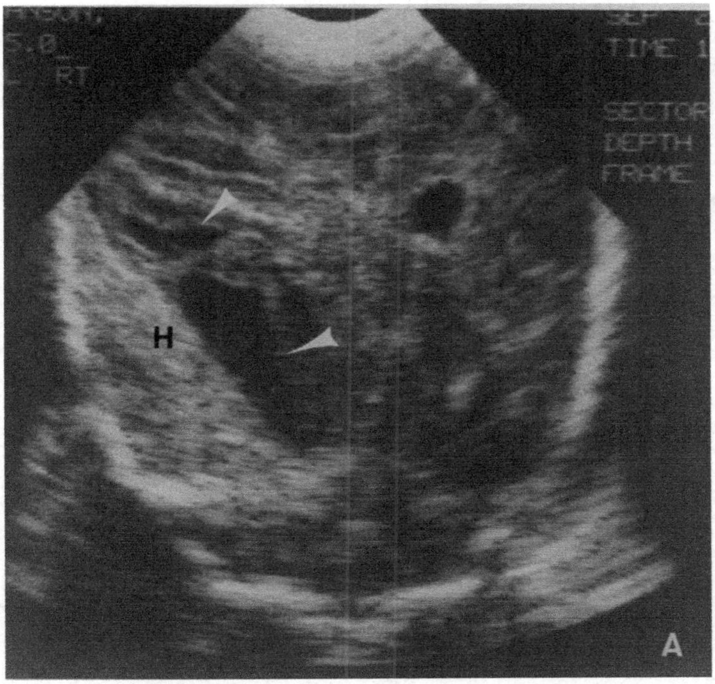


Fig. 3 A

Fig. 3. Acute subdural hematoma. A) Coronal, B) Right parasagittal, and C) Left parasagittal scans demonstrate large subdural hematoma (*H*), partially echogenic and partially liquefied displacing brain (arrowheads) and midline structures from right to left. Right lateral ventricle is compressed. Right temporal lobe (*T*) and Sylvian fissure (curved arrow) are elevated by hematoma. Autopsy confirmed large right subdural hematoma

respiratory distress. In the presence of the signs, rapid diagnosis and surgical management may be essential for survival and prevention of permanent neurologic sequelae. Ultrasonography may provide the most expeditious means of determining the site of the subdural hematoma or appropriate surgical intervention.

Sonography of an acute subdural hematoma shows displacement of the brain away from the bony calvarium by the hematoma which is usually echogenic in the acute stage, but may be partially sonolucent and liquefied. Fig. 2 is a 6 month old who was hit in the head with a brick. Coronal scans show echogenic hematoma in the interhemispheric fissure and separating the gyri of the brain from the fontanelle and the bony calvarium. Extraaxial fluid collections are often best visualized on magnified views of the interhemispheric fissure and the brain immediately under the fontanelle (Fig. 2 B). The extensive scalp edema present results in reverberation artifacts which impede visualization of the intracranial contents. Sub-

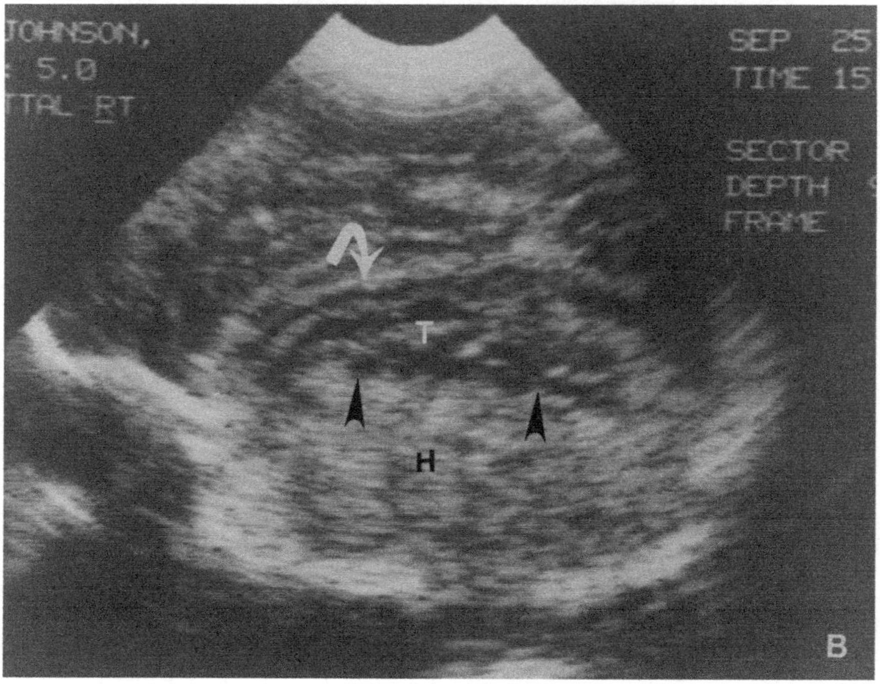
JOHNSON,
5.0
TTAL RT
SEP 25
TIME 15
SECTOR
DEPTH
FRAME
T
H
B

Fig. 3 B

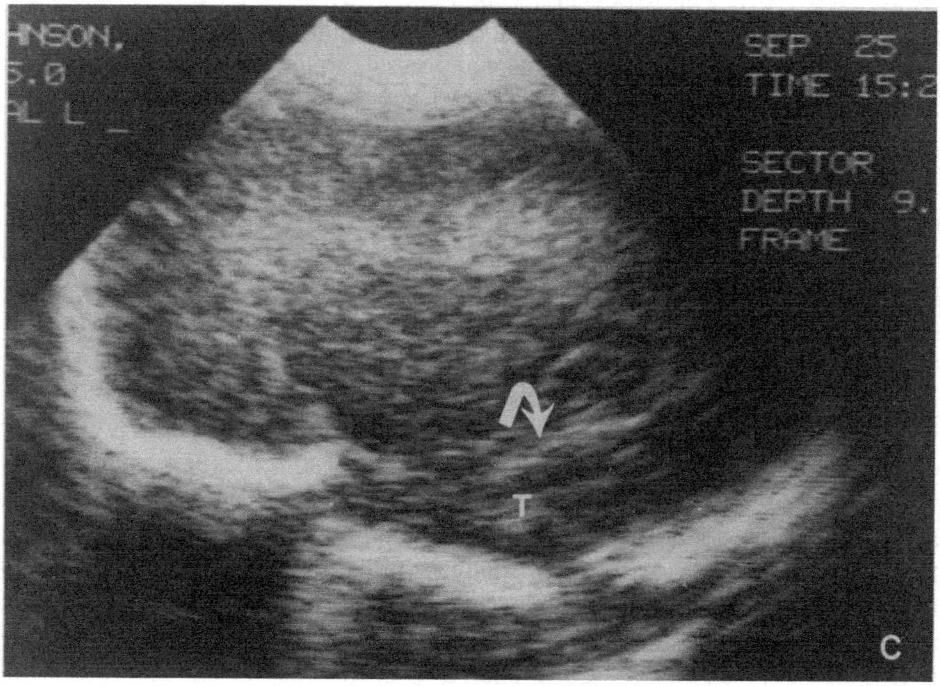
HNSON,
5.0
AL L
SEP 25
TIME 15:2
SECTOR
DEPTH 9.
FRAME
T
C

Fig. 3 C

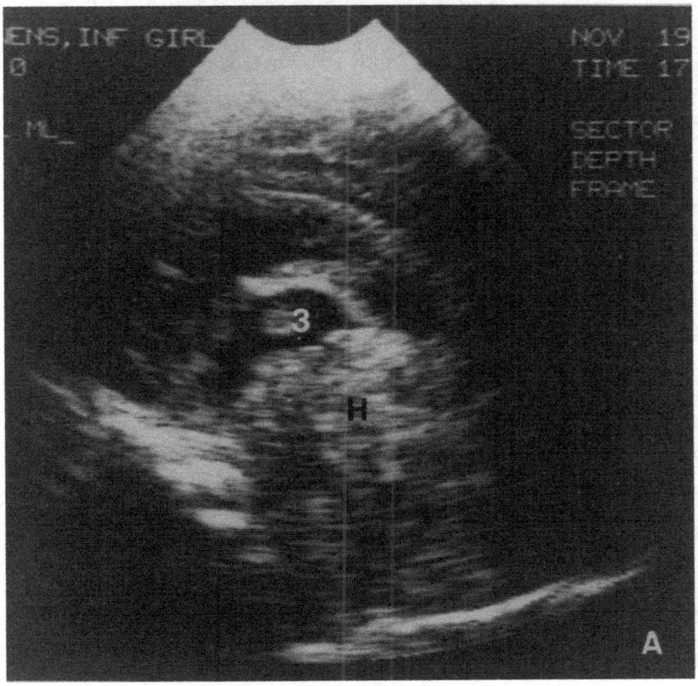


Fig. 4 A

Fig. 4. Posterior fossa hemorrhage. Term infant with seizures, abnormal cry, and decreased motion of extremities. A) Midline sagittal and B) Modified coronal sonograms demonstrate mild dilatation of lateral (*V*) and third (*3*) ventricles. Posterior fossa structures usually visible are obliterated by echogenic hematoma (*H*) which bulges upwards through the tent, displacing the third ventricle. C) and D) CT scans show extensive posterior fossa hemorrhage with subdural and cerebellar involvement. Blood extends superiorly through incisura into region of ambient wing and quadrigeminal plate cisterns. Despite evacuation of posterior fossa hematoma, patient died and autopsy demonstrated a lacerated left tentorium, likely the site of hemorrhage

arachnoid hemorrhage may also be detected[5], though it may be difficult to distinguish from a subdural collection.

Another patient (Fig. 3) has a large acute subdural hematoma over the right parietal and temporal lobes. The hematoma is partially echogenic due to clotted blood, but some parts are liquified and sonolucent. The surface of the brain is significantly displaced away from the bony calvarium. The midline is shifted, and the ipsilateral ventricle is compressed. The subtemporal portion of the hematoma displaces the Sylvian fissure upward.

Fig. 4 is a one day old term infant with a seizure, abnormal cry, and decreased motion of the extremities. The spinal tap was bloody. Sonography shows obliteration of the normal posterior fossa structures by a

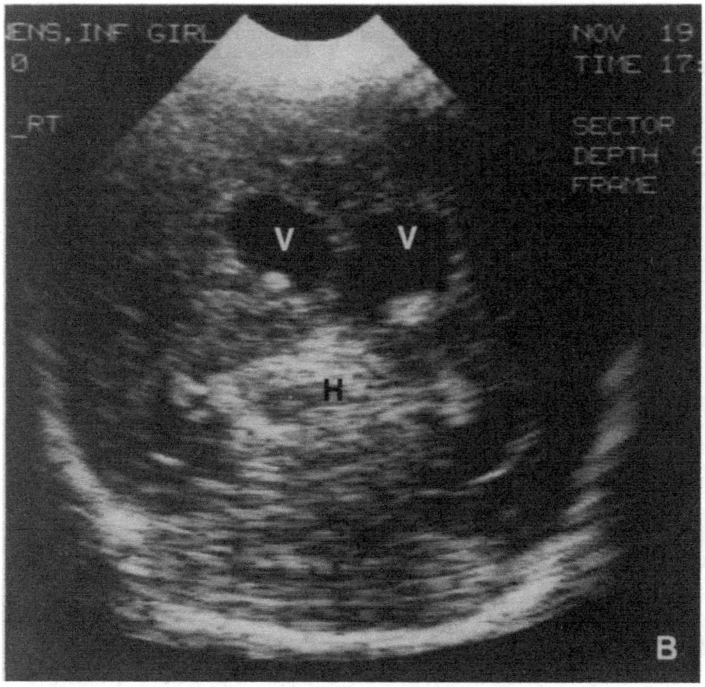


Fig. 4 B

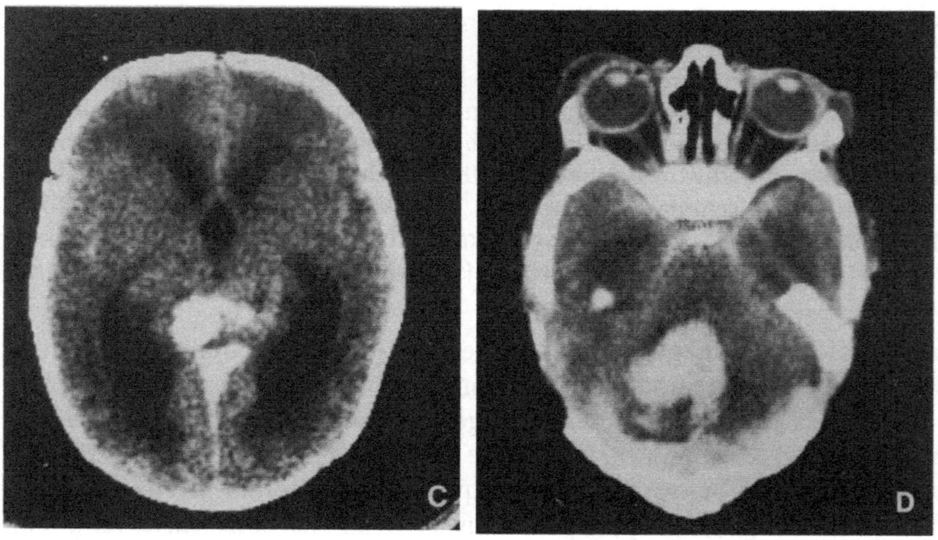


Fig. 4 C–D

hemorrhage which is both subdural and within the posterior fossa brain itself. The blood is echogenic and obliterates the normal anatomy. The lateral and third ventricles are moderately dilated as well. The echogenic mass in the posterior fossa bulges up through the tent and displaces the third ventricle.

Posterior fossa hemorrhages may not be recognized on sonography unless the normal structures readily imaged with current equipment are carefully studied[9].

### *4.2. Chronic*

Although acute subdural hematomas may occur in the neonatal period, they are not as frequently seen as chronic subdural hematomas which occur later during infancy. Subdural accumulations may also result from meningitis, but true chronic hematomas are almost invariably traumatic in origin. The accumulation consists of blood-tinged xanthochromic high protein fluid, usually bilaterally. The traumatic episode responsible for such hematomas is frequently difficult to define. It is assumed, however, that such hematomas probably occur as a consequence of infant abuse in many instances.

The clinical presentation is usually related to intracranial hypertension and to cortical irritation. Thus, the presenting features include macrocrania, increased fontanelle tension, irritability, vomiting and, frequently, seizures. Retinal hemorrhages are found in approximately 50% of patients.

Ultrasonography has been a very useful diagnostic tool in the management of infants with chronic subdural hematomas. The diagnosis can usually be established easily and the extent of the effusion can be determined. Bilateral echolucent spaces are seen between the cranial vault and the underlying compressed cortex (Fig. 5). Sonography also is useful in determining ventricular size as this is significant in prognosis. Our experience has indicated that, if there is ventricular enlargement in combination with subdural hematomas, the prognosis for normal development is quite low. Ultrasonography has also proven to be a very useful and easy means of following the progressive decrease of subdural fluid and reexpansion of the brain during the course of treatment by subdural tapping.

Fig. 6 shows a patient with a left fronto-parietal subdural fluid collection which is readily visualized on CT but could not be identified on ultrasound because of its location high over the convexity in an area which could not be imaged through the fontanelle. The baby is 11 months old and the fontanelle has started to close so that the peripheral brain is not imaged. This problem increases as the fontanelle gets smaller. Scans through the parietal bone can be performed although these also decrease in diagnostic quality as the bone gets thicker with age.

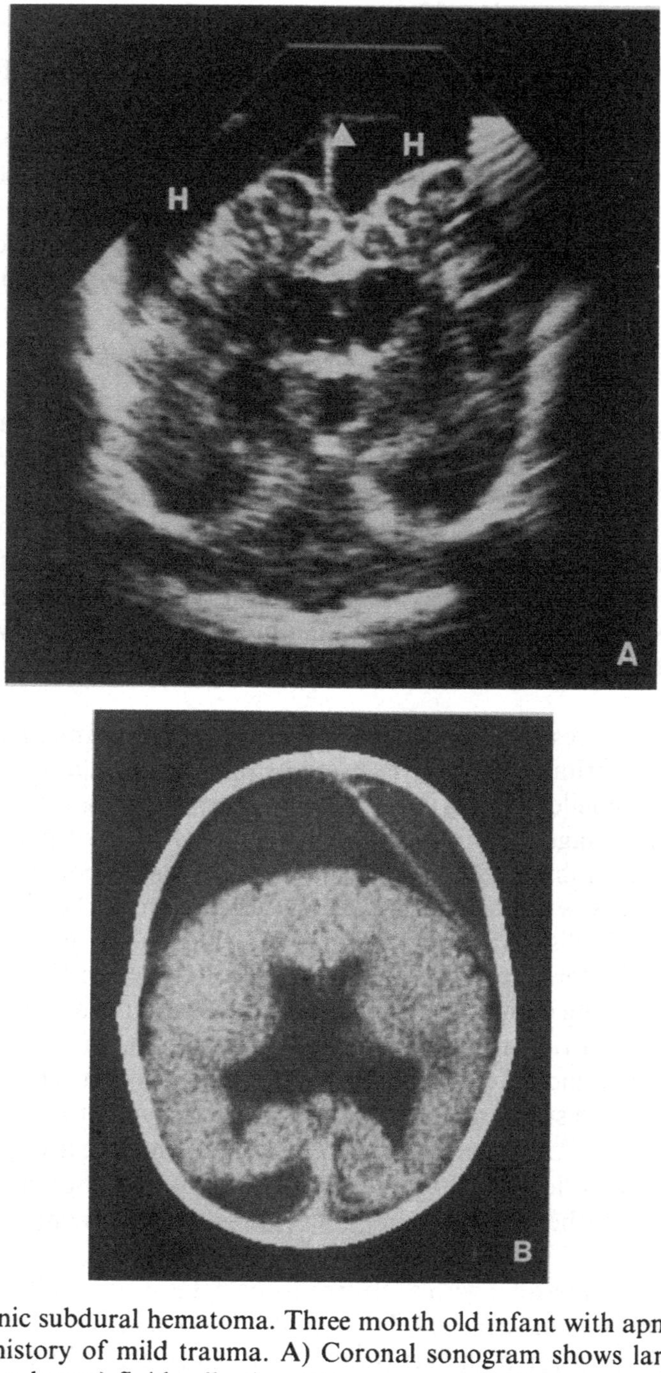


Fig. 5. Chronic subdural hematoma. Three month old infant with apnea episodes and recent history of mild trauma. A) Coronal sonogram shows large bilateral subdural (sonolucent) fluid collection (*H*) separating cerebral cortex from cranial vault. Falx cerebri (arrowhead) seen as linear midline structure outlined by fluid. Ventricles are moderately enlarged. B) CT scan two years later shows chronic subdural fluid collections, enlarged ventricles, and brain atrophy. Patient is severely mentally retarded with seizure disorder. (A: reproduced with permission from DS Babcock and BK Han: Radiology 139: 665–676, 1981)

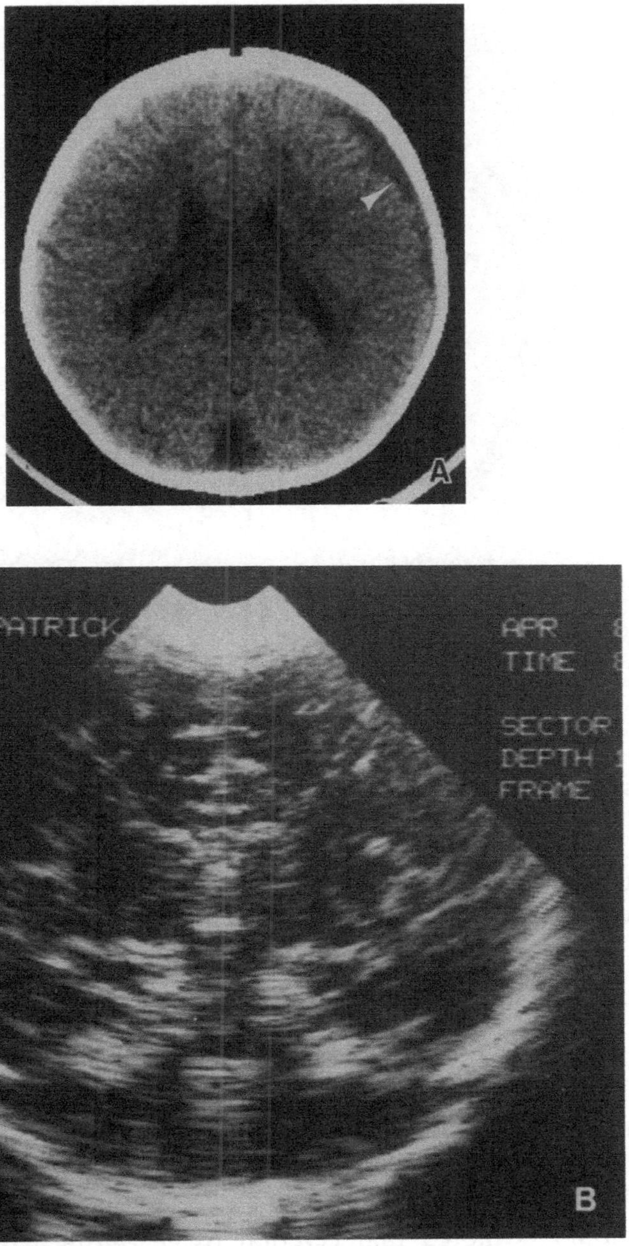


Fig. 6. Localized subdural fluid not visualized on ultrasound. A) CT scan shows localized fronto-parietal subdural fluid collection (arrow) high over the convexity. B) Coronal sonogram fails to demonstrate the fluid because of peripheral location in "blind spot". As fontanelle closes, the peripheral brain over the convexity is less well imaged

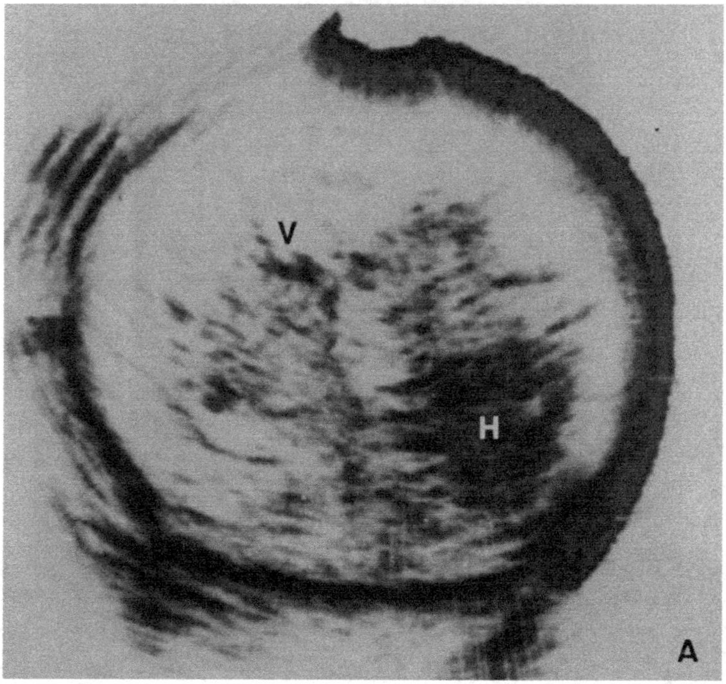


Fig. 7 A

Fig. 7. Intracerebral hemorrhage. Full-term infant with seizure. A) Coronal sonogram demonstrates echogenic mass in left temporal region representing acute intraparenchymal hematoma (*H*). Lateral ventricle (*V*) is minimally dilated. B) Axial CT scan without contrast shows temporal lobe mass with increased density compatible with intracerebral hematoma. C) Follow-up axial sonogram shows large porencephalic cyst (*C*) in area of previous hematoma. Lateral ventricles (*V*) now moderately dilated

## 5. Intraparenchymal Hemorrhage

Traumatic intraparenchymal hemorrhage is relatively rare during infancy. The most common cause of intracerebral hemorrhage is that which results from germinal matrix hemorrhage in premature infants. This, however, is not traumatic in origin.

It should be noted that cerebral tissue during early infancy reacts differently to impact than in older ages. It is believed that myelin is the principal factor in determining brain compliance to mechanical trauma. Since myelinization is far from complete at the time of birth, the response of cerebral tissue to mechanical stress is quite different than the response at a later age. Stress to the head sufficient to cause damage to cerebral tissue results in "tears" in the white matter rather than the contusion and hemorrhage most often found beyond early infancy. The tears result in

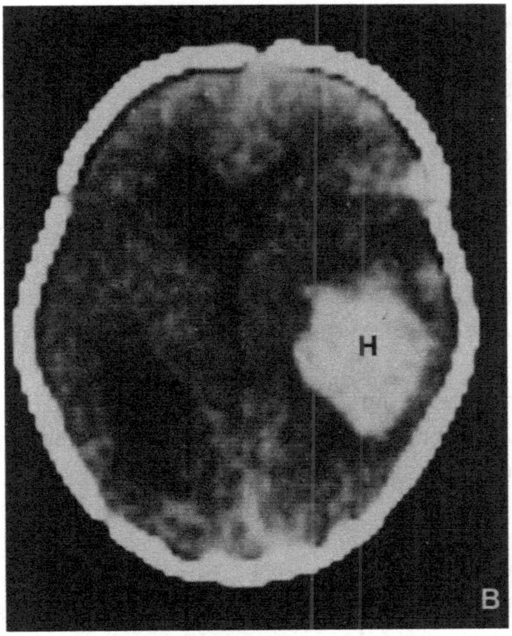


Fig. 7 B

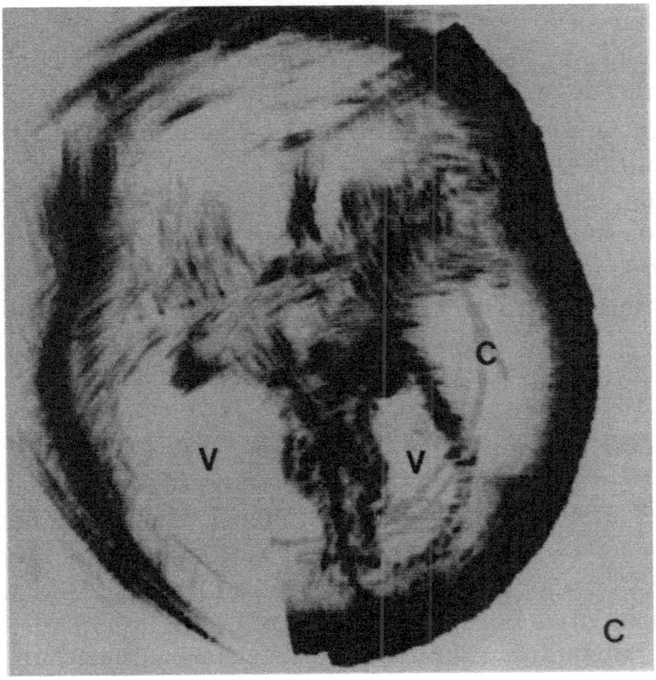


Fig. 7 C

cavities which may contain blood initially and, later, become smooth walled glial-lined excavations. These cavities rarely involve the cortex and it is believed that apparent cortical contusions may be the consequence of ischemia rather than trauma.

Concerning impact injuries in older infants, Courville found from autopsy observations that there was considerable difference in the frequency of contracoup cerebral injuries after trauma[4]. Contracoup damage occurred in only 10% of children under 3 years of age and progressively increased to approximately 85% in fatal injuries to adults. Pliability of the skull and compliance of the cerebral tissue are believed again to be relevant to this difference.

Intracerebellar hemorrhage has also been noted to occur with some frequency in low birth weight infants[6]. The mechanism of hemorrhage is not clear, but may be related to pathophysiologic mechanisms similar to those occurring in germinal matrix hemorrhage. In term infants, however, cerebellar hemorrhage may be a direct consequence of mechanical pressure. The risk factors include maternal (e.g., small birth canal), fetal (e.g., large head), labor (e.g., precipitous), and delivery (e.g., breech) factors. The same type of occipital compression which may result in dural and sinus tears may also presumably lead to cerebellar hemorrhage. Because of its strategic location in relation to cerebrospinal fluid circulation and to the brain stem, it is imperative that such hemorrhage be suspected on clinical ground, verified by neuroimaging techniques, and promptly treated surgically. Conservative therapy has been successful in rare instances. It is noteworthy, however, that poor neurologic outcome is more common after cerebellar than after cerebral hemorrhage[12].

Intracerebral and intracerebellar hematomas are echogenic in the acute phase (Fig. 7) and usually more echogenic than adjacent brain. As the hematoma resolves, it becomes less echogenic and eventually liquifies resulting in an area of porencephaly[1]. This process takes weeks to months.

## 6. Conclusion

Ultrasonography may be of assistance in screening newborns and infants for intracranial trauma and for following the resulution of hematomas. It has certain advantages over CT scanning, such as availability in the nursery, lower cost, and lack of radiation to the developing brain. The principal disadvantages are lack of resolution in defining intracranial structures and some limitation of visualizing surface lesions in the high parietal region. For these reasons, ultrasonography should not be considered as a substitute for CT scanning, but rather as an adjunctive diagnostic method.

## References


1. Babcock DS, Han BK (1981) Cranial ultrasonography of infants. Williams and Wilkins, Baltimore, pp 194–225
2. Blank NK, Strad R, Gilles FH, Palakshappa A (1978) Posterior fossa subdural hematomas in neonates. Arch Neurol 35: 108–111
3. Choux M (1986) Extracerebral hematomas in children. In: Vigouroux RP, McLaurin RL (eds) Advances in neurotraumatology, vol 1: Extracerebral collections. Springer, Wien New York, pp 173–208
4. Courville CB (1965) Contrecoup injuries of the brain in infancy. Arch Surg 90: 157–165
5. Ennis MG, Kaude JV, Williams JL (1985) Sonographic diagnosis of subarachnoid hemorrhage in premature newborn infants: a retrospective study with histopathologic and CT correlation. J Ultrasound Med 4: 183–187
6. Martin R, Roessman U, Fanaroff A (1976) Massive intracerebellar hemorrhage in low-birth-weight infants. J Pediatr 89: 290–293
7. Mazza C, Pasqualin G, Feriotti G, DaPian R (1982) Traumatic extradural hematomas in children: experience with 62 cases. Acta Neurochir (Wien) 65: 67–80
8. McLaurin RL (1985) Subdural hematomas in children. In: Wilkins RH, Rengachary SS (eds) Neurosurgery. McGraw-Hill Book Co, New York, pp 2211–2214
9. Reeder JD, Setzer ES, Kaude JV (1982) Ultrasonographic detection of perinatal intracerebellar hemorrhage. Pediatrics 70: 385–386
10. Rumack CM, Johnson ML (1984) Perinatal and infant brain imaging: role of ultrasound and computed tomography. Yearbook Medical Publishers, Chicago, pp 117–153
11. Shapiro K (ed) (1983) Pediatric head trauma. Futura Publishing Co Ind, Mt Kisko New York
12. Williams WD, Percy AK, Fishman MA, Cheek WR, Desmond MM, LaFevers N, Thurber SD (1985) Cerebellar hemorrhage in the term neonate: developmental and neurologic outcome. Pediatr Neurol 1: 356–360

# Drug Protection for Head Injuries

F. MURILLO, M. A. MUÑOZ, and P. ALBERT

Seville (Spain)

**Contents**



High dosage barbiturates to reduce intracranial pressure which is resistant to osmotic agents were first successfully employed by Ishii[1]. Since that time, interest in this new method has increased. Its clinical use has expanded in recent years and there have been many important papers written not only about the effectiveness of barbiturates in lowering intracranial pressure[2–5] but of their value in improving the outcome of patients suffering from head injuries[6–8]. As the use of this therapeutic method has spread, so has the controversy as to its ability to reduce mortality and morbidity.

As a result of the doubts raised by Miller[9], other authors have begun to question the effectiveness of barbiturates in treating head injuries. They have expressed doubts as to the very foundations which its supporters have stressed: reduction of intracranial pressure (ICP) not responsive to less aggressive conventional treatment, decrease in edema formation[10] and outcome improvement. Before setting down our experience in the use of high dosage barbiturates in the treatment of head injury patients, we would like to make some observations.

## 1. Importance of ICP Control in Severe Head Injury

The practice of continuous recording of ICP has made us aware that a large number of patients with severe head injuries suffer from some degree of intracranial hypertension. The percentages that have been published as to its incidence have oscillated from 30% to 60%[11–15]. Greater attention paid to early diagnosis, treatment of hypoxia and of arterial hypotension, immediately after injury, seems to meet with a decrease in the prevalence of intracranial hypertension. However, a number of patients have been observed in whom conventional methods to reduce ICP have failed. These patients fall into the group of severe head-injured patients who suffer from malignant or uncontrollable intracranial hypertension. This select group constitutes 15% of the patients admitted to our series. Similar percentages have been reported by other authors. Miller *et al.*[16] reported uncontrolled intracranial hypertension in 16% of their patients. Rea and Rockswold[7] found this complication in 13% and Marshall *et al.*[15] encountered a somewhat higher percentage (16%) in their patients.

The mortality rate in patients with malignant intracranial hypertension is unacceptably high. Miller *et al.*[11, 15] have documented a mortality rate of 92% in patients with ICP greater than 20 mm Hg. McGraw and his colleagues[17] found a 100% mortality rate in head-injured patients with an ICP average of more than 30 mm Hg throughout the monitoring period. Byrnes and Ducker[18] reported a mortality rate of 84% in patients whose ICP level was higher than 25 mm Hg.

Although the injurious effect on the brain of raised ICP is not direct, but is a result of cerebral ischemia or brain shift and distortion[5, 9, 19] the control of high ICP continues to be a major objective in the treatment of patients with severe brain injuries[20]. Many advances have been made in the management of these patients. The CT scanner allows an improved and quicker evacuation of expansive processes. The neurological intensive care units provide painstaking vigilance of these patients. They are meticulously treated with steroids, osmotic agents, cerebrospinal fluid (CSF) drainage and hyperventilation. Nevertheless, in spite of all our endeavors, there is still an excessive number of patients who die due to malignant intracranial hypertension. Therefore, a search has been undertaken to look for new methods to stop these unnecessary deaths and barbiturate treatment may be the solution.

## 2. Role of High Dosage Barbiturates in Posttrauma Intracranial Hypertension

Many studies, mainly experimental, have stressed the potential benefits that barbiturates offer in the way of protection from brain ischemia following stroke, cardiac arrest and other forms of global ischemia[21–23]. In severe head injuries, diminished cerebral blood flow and consumption of oxygen is frecuently encountered[24, 25]. However, the use of barbiturates has been focussed on the reduction of raised ICP along with the preservation of the cerebral perfusion pressure (CPP).

Although the actual mechanisms by which barbiturates reduce ICP remain unknown, there is strong evidence that they increase the cerebrovascular resistance and thereby reduce the cerebral blood volume. Therefore, barbiturates by decreasing ICP and increasing CPP could improve the cerebral blood flow. It is still not known if this occurs in both damaged and normal tissue[12]. Allman *et al.*[26] have stated that rapid reduction in ICP after barbiturate anesthesia could possibly be due to the increase in serum osmolality that such agents induce. Reduction in vasogenic edema formation, which frequently develops in head-injured patients, is another of the potential benefits that barbiturates offer. In experimental cortical lesions, induced by freezing techniques (cryogenic), barbiturates have been shown to reduce the development of cerebral edema[10, 27]. This reduction is possibly due to an increase in the cerebral arteriolar resistances and a fall in the capillary hydrostatic pressure in the damaged areas of the brain. The attraction of free radicals of oxygen so that endothelial damage can be prevented is another of the mechanisms that have been called upon to reduce vasogenic edema formation[28]. Marsh *et al.*[12] think that a reduction in the absolute blood pressure level as well as the fluctuations in arterial pressure caused by painful stimuli can have an effect on the prevention of edema formation.

These benefits, some theoretical and others proven, are a result of the administration of barbiturates in patients with high ICP, but have still not been sufficient to dispel doubts concerning the effectiveness of the use of this method in applied medicine. This is not only true in the treatment of malignant intracranial hypertension but also in the improvement of the prognosis of these patients[9]; more so if one takes into consideration the potential risks that the use of barbiturates involves.

Recent tests carried out in the United States have suggested that the use of high dosage barbiturates will improve the outcome of patients with severe head injuries[29]. Sidi *et al.*[20] have proposed that barbiturate administration in severe head injuries is associated with decreased mortality. The beneficial effects of barbiturates in ICP control and outcome were reported in previous publications by Rockoff *et al.*[3], Saul *et al.*[4] and Marshall *et al.*[5]. However, since barbiturates could possibly have increased the percentage of patients having intracranial hypertension resistant to conventional therapy, Miller[9] has raised some questions about this new therapeutic step. Whereas 25% of the patients in the San Diego series[5] in which barbiturates were administered had uncontrollable hypertension, the percentage in the Richmond series[30] in which barbiturates were not used was only 16%.

From a group of 210 patients with severe head injuries, Rea and Rockswold[7] separated a group of 27 patients (13%) who had intracranial hypertension that was resistant to treatment. This sub-group was treated with steroids, hyperventilation, mannitol, surgical decompression, restriction of fluids and the head of the bed was raised, as indicated. Although mortality rates close to 100% in this type of uncontrollable intracranial hypertension have been reported, this sub-group treated by Rea and Rockswold[7], had ICP levels normalized in 56% of the patients and the mortality rate was 52%. Norby and Nesbakken[8] have reported a controlled clinical study of two groups of patients with severe head injuries. Both groups were similar in age, type of lesion according to the CT scanner, Glasgow Coma Score (GCS), pupillary reactions and associated lesions. In the group treated with high dosages of thiopental, an appreciable difference as far as ICP control and reduction of morbidity/mortality was found.

Our experience with high dosage barbiturates can also be considered satisfactory[31]. In a group of 185 consecutive head-injured patients (GCS lower than 8) admitted to our hospital, 28 patients had resistant intracranial hypertension. This sub-group had an ICP level greater than 25 mm Hg for longer than half an hour, following adequate resuscitation, evacuation of lesions as indicated and having employed maximum postural hyperventilation and mannitol or glycerol. Since extradural monitoring was instituted, none of the patients underwent CSF drainage and no ventricular catheters were used. The barbiturate chosen was thiopental and it was administered in an initial "shock" dosage of 1.5 milligram/kilo of weight and the maintenance dosage was given in a continuous perfusion of between 3–6 milligrams/kilo of weight/hour. The characteristics of the 28 patients are shown in Table 1.

After 36 hours of continuous thiopental infusion, 39.28% of this sub-group had an ICP level lower than 20 mm Hg. The mortality rate was 35.71% (10 patients). One patient remained in a vegetative state and another was found to be severely disabled a year after injury. Good functional results were shown by the other 16 patients (57.1%). It should be pointed out that all of the deaths occurred in patients whose ICP did not descend with the barbiturate infusion. Table 2 shows the ICP levels of these

*Table 1*

| | |
|---|---|
| Average age | 32.6 years |
| Unreactive pupils | 10.07% |
| Decerebrate/Flaccid | 32.14% |
| Surgical mass lesion | 67.85% |

*Table 2*

| ICP mm Hg | Good recovery | Moderately disabled | Severely disabled | Vege- tative | Dead |
|---|---|---|---|---|---|
| 0–20 | 7 | 4 | 0 | 0 | 0 |
| 21–30 | 2 | 3 | 1 | 1 | 0 |
| 31–40 | 0 | 0 | 0 | 0 | 1 |
| 40– | 0 | 0 | 0 | 0 | 9 |

patients after 36 hours of thiopental infusion and the results a year after injury.

We believe that the results we obtained in these patients with malignant intracranial hypertension speak out in favor of the use of barbiturates in those patients whose ICP has not become normal after energetic resuscitation and the use of less aggressive methods of proven utility.

### 3. Considerations on the Use of High Dosage Barbiturates

The number of potential risks intrinsic in barbiturate therapy makes it necessary to keep strict vigilance over the patients in a well-equipped intensive care unit by a highly-trained staff. We believe that the lack of these conditions has contributed to keeping the controversy alive, whether to use or not to use barbiturates, and has offered its detractors arguments against this therapy.

Barbiturate therapy has two principal pitfalls. One is the loss of neurological contact with the patient and the other is the risk of arterial hypotension. An additional difficulty is the lack of a satisfactory method of adjusting the effectiveness of barbiturate dosages, since blood levels are very poor indicators of barbiturate concentration in brain tissue and CSF[32]. Another problem is that continuous monitoring of an electroencephalogram is not available in many intensive care units. In our experience, the only guideline employed in barbiturate dosages given has been the ICP response and the hemodynamic tolerance[31]. The loss of neurological contact requires perceptive ICP monitoring as well as serial CT scan studies. Multi-method evoked-potentials seem to be of use in following the evolution of patients in barbiturate coma[21, 33]. The danger of arterial hypotension makes it necessary to continuously monitor the arterial pressure, the central venous pressure and frequently, the pulmonary arterial wedge pressure by means of a Swan-Ganz catheter. Together with these hemodynamic controls, periodic analyses of the blood pH and gases as well as the albumin level or colloidosmotic pressure in plasma are necessary. We have observed that there is a diminished incidence of dangerous arterial hypotension by administering barbiturates in continuous infusion rather than in a bolus. In our series of 28 patients with malignant intracranial hypertension only 3 patients had a mean arterial pressure (MAP) lower than 80 torr after barbiturate infusion. We feel that there is less risk of cardiocirculatory depression if barbiturates are administered in a continuous infusion and that this allows for a more secure management of the patient.

To sum up, we think that barbiturate therapy has a place in the treatment of traumatic intracranial hypertension that is resistant to less aggressive conventional methods. Nevertheless, its obvious risks make meticulous, follow-up clinical studies necessary in order to define the future role of barbiturates in the protection of these head-injured patients.

## References

1. Ishii S (1966) Brain swelling: Studies of structural, physiologic and biochemical alterations. In: Caveness WF, Walker AE (eds) Head injury. JB Lippincott, Philadelphia, pp 276–283
2. Shapiro HM, Wyte SR, Loeser J (1974) Barbiturate-augmented hypothermia for reduction of persisten intracranial hypertension. J Neurosurg 40: 90–100
3. Rockoff MA, Marshall LF, Shapiro HM (1979) High-dose barbiturate therapy in humans: A clinical review of 60 patients. Ann Neurol 6: 194–199
4. Saul TG, Ducker TB (1982) Effect of intracranial pressure monitoring and aggressive treatment on mortality in severe head injury. J Neurosurg 56: 498–503
5. Marshall LF, Smith RW, Shapiro HM (1979) The outcome with aggressive treatment in severe head injuries. Part II: acute and chronic barbiturate administration in the management of head injury. J Neurosurg 50: 26–30
6. Muñoz Sanchez MA, Murillo Cabezas F, Morales Ramos F, Ruano del Campo JJ, Albert Lasierra P (1983) Nuestra experiencia en el tratamiento del traumatismo craneoencefálico grave. Medicina Intensiva 7: 80–86
7. Rea GL, Rockswold GL (1983) Barbiturate therapy in uncontrolled intracranial hypertension. Neurosurg 12: 401–404
8. Nordby HK, Nesbakken R (1984) The effect of high-dose barbiturate descompression after severe head injury. A controlled clinical trial. Acta Neurochir (Wien) 72: 157–166
9. Miller JD (1979) Barbiturates and raised intracranial pressure. Ann Neurol 3: 189–193
10. Smith AL, Margue JJ (1976) Anesthetics and cerebral edema. Anesthesiology 45: 64–72
11. Miller JD, Ward JD, Becker DP *et al* (1979) Significance of intracranial hypertension in severe head injury. J Neurosurg 47: 503–516
12. Marsh ML, Marshall LF, Shapiro HM (1977) Neurosurgical intensive care. Anesthesiology 47: 149–163

13. Murillo Cabezas F, Muñoz Sanchez MA, Morales Ramos F *et al* (1981) Interès de la monitorización intracraneal en cuidados intensivos. Medicina Intensiva 1: 480–484
14. Bellegarige R, Ducker TB (1983) Control of intracranial pressure in severe head injury. In: Ishii S, Nagai H, Brock M (eds) Intracranial pressure V. Springer, Berlin Heidelberg New York Tokyo, pp 567–571
15. Narayan RK, Kishore PR, Becker DP *et al* (1982) To monitor or not to monitor? A review of our experience with severe head injury. J Neurosurg 56: 650–659
16. Miller JD, Butterworth JF, Gudeman SK *et al* (1981) Further experience in the management of sever head injury. J Neurosurg 54: 289–299
17. McGraw CP, Howard G, O'Connor C (1983) Outcome associated with management based on ICP monitoring. In: Ishii S, Nagai H, Brock M (eds) Intracranial pressure V. Springer, Berlin Heidelberg New York Tokyo, pp 558–561
18. Byrnes DP, Ducker TB (1980) Continuous measurement of intracranial pressure in 127 severe head injuries. In: Shulman K, Marmarov A, Miller JD *et al* (eds) Intracranial pressure IV. Springer, Berlin Heidelberg New York, pp 73–78
19. Langfitt TW (1969) Increased intracranial pressure. Clin Neurosurg 16: 436–471
20. Sidi A, Coteus, Hadani M *et al* (1983) Long-term barbiturate infusion to reduce intracranial pressure. Crit Care Med 11: 478–481
21. Safar P, Stezoski W, Nemoto EM (1976) Ameloration of brain damage after 12 minutes of cardiac arrest in dogs. Arch Neurol 33: 91–95
22. Smith AL, Hoft JT, Nielsen SL *et al* (1975) Barbiturate protection from cerebral infarction in primates. Stroke 6: 28–33
23. Bleyaert AL, Nemoto EM, Stezoski H *et al* (1976) Thiopental therapy after 16 minutes of global brain ischemia. Crit Care Med 4: 130–131
24. Hass WK (1976) Prognosic value of cerebral oxidative metabolism in head trauma. Head injuries. McLaurin RL (ed) Second Chicago Symposium on Neurol Traum. Grune and Stratton, New York, pp 35–37
25. Obrist W, Langfitt TW, Jaggi JC, Cruz J, Gennarelli TA (1984) Cerebral flow and metabolism in comatose patients with acute head injury. Relationship to intracranial hypertension. J Neurosurg 61: 241–253
26. Allman FD, Talamo J, Rogers MC (1980) Increased serum osmolality following pentobarbital anesthesia. A possible mechanism for lowering ICP. Annual scientific and educational symposium of the society of Critical Care Medicine (Abstracts) Crit Care Med 2: 27
27. Clasen RA, Pandolfi S, Casey D (1974) Furosemide and pentobarbital in cryogenic cerebral injury and edema. Neurology (Minneap) 24: 642–648
28. Siesjö BK, Carlsson C, Hägerdal M, Nordstrom CH (1976) Brain metabolism in the critically ill. Crit Care Med 4: 283–294
29. Marshall LF (1985) Reduction of brain damage: fantasy, reality and pitfalls. Proceedings of the 4th World Congress on Intensive and Critical Care Medicine, Jerusalem 1985, pp 206–208
30. Becker DP, Miller JD, Ward JD *et al* (1977) The outcome from severe head

injury with early diagnosis and intensive management. J Neurosurg 47: 491–502

31. Murillo Cabezas F, Muñoz Sanchez MA, Dominguez Roldán JM, Ruano del Campo JJ, Gonzalez Menendez E, Albert P (1986) Barbitúricos a altas dosis en la hipertensión endocraneal incontrolable. Medicina Intensiva 10: 164–168
32. Bruce DA, Gennarelli TA, Langfitt TW (1978) Resuscitation from coma due to head injury. Crit Care Med 6: 254–269
33. Chaparro P, Muñoz MA, Madrazo J, Ruano JJ, Murillo F (1984) Potenciales evocados en el TCE grave. Medicina Intensiva 8: 247–252

# Epilogue

There is no doubt that serious injuries to the spine are one of the major and most devastating health care problems that besets man, affecting so many body systems and necessitating the involvement of so many medical, public services and other specialists. The patient's whole life may quite suddenly become disrupted with possible permanent personal, family, educational and employment problems.

The appreciation, organization and harnessing of proper resources for traumatic paraplegic patients is indeed a very real challenge, and the study and management of serious spinal trauma is a microcosm of the overall scientific and humanitarian progress of man.

The aim in this, the second volume in the "Advances of Neurotraumatology" series under the auspices of the International Neurotraumatology Committee (of the World Federation of Neurosurgical Societies) whose Chairman is Professor Robert P. Vigouroux, and Deputy Chairman myself, is set out in the Foreword to volume I, and readers will have read this. In the Foreword for the second volume of the series, Professor Vigouroux gives an outline of the contents of this book. The policy of the series is to give each author, or group of authors free reign to express his or her subject.

There is no intention whatsoever to attempt to produce a text-book on "Thoracic and Lumbar Spine and Spinal Cord Injuries"; each invited contributor is a specialist of international repute in the particular topic of his presentation. The subject matters are individual and personal, there are no cross-references, and there is no attempt to be comprehensive. Thus there are understandably, from the Managing Editor's viewpoint, some obvious and important omissions, including the very important matter of prevention, and of prehospital management, and there is insufficient stress on the importance of having specialized spinal paralysis services which are an integral part of a general hospital of excellence with all vital facilities for the modern essential investigations and comprehensive management of such patients, about 30% of whom will have a significant associated injury. Possibly a chapter should have been devoted to "Functional Electrical Stimulation" in the spinal paralyzed patient, but we require to be practical and selective in all books of this form to limit the scope of contents to keep the book of reasonable size and price.

Pathophysiological aspects are only briefly touched upon, and no attempt in this volume has been made to discuss such important aspects of research such as attempts to achieve spinal cord regeneration. Experimental studies are confined to the somewhat controversial work on the possible therapeutic value of what is called "revascularization of the traumatized spinal cord"; a new procedure which is under critical review by several independent workers.

It is in the sphere of patient management that there is always the greatest controversy regarding spinal trauma, but we have been fortunate in obtaining valuable contributions from distinguished doctors, one a French neurosurgeon, Dr. Reynier, who is not adverse to carrying out a spinal operation for many of his patients with thoracic, thoraco-lumbar, or lumbar injuries; and the other, almost contrary view of the so-called "conservative approach" which is clearly set out by doctors Frankel, Masri, and Ravichandran. Your editors are very pleased to have these important viewpoints; suffice to say that the Managing Editor is a "conservative neurosurgeon" with (probably well known) published views on the indications, merits and demerits of various investigations and therapies for such patients. However, both the clinical aspects of these patients and their nonspinal but other operative treatments, rehabilitation and outcome of expert management are clearly enunciated in this book.

As was decided when this series was envisaged, each volume will contain one or more sections outwith the main theme of the book, to take the opportunity of referring to current, different neurotraumatological topics and "Sonography of Traumatic Cranial Haemorrhage", and "Drug Protection for Head Injuries" were chosen for this particular volume.

In conclusion, one would quote from Tolstoy, in his book "War and Peace" (and "neurotraumatology" can be considered a battle as such); he stated: "The most difficult but most essential thing is to love life, but to love it even when one suffers because life is all."

The editors have the greatest pleasure in thanking all the contributors for their interest and active cooperation and for their forebearance regarding editorial recommendations. We feel and hope that their efforts have not been in vain in contributing to a book devoted to such an important practical medical subject, where the aim is to provide even better care for our spinal-injured patients.

At all times the publishers, Messrs. Springer-Verlag, Vienna, have been most helpful and encouraging and have done their best to keep all of us to deadlines. On the behalf of all concerned with writing this book I offer them our thanks and good wishes.

Phillip Harris, F.R.C.S.E., F.R.C.P.E.,
F.R.C.S. (Glas.), F.R.S.E.
Edinburgh, Scotland

# Subject Index

# Modern Concepts in Neurotraumatology

Edited by

**S. Lindgren,** Professor of Neurosurgery, Department of Neurosurgery, Sahlgren's Hospital, Göteborg, Sweden

1986. 65 figures. VIII, 159 pages.
Soft cover DM 170,–, öS 1190,–. ISBN 3-211-81931-2
Reduced price for subscribers to "Acta Neurochirurgica":
Soft cover DM 153,–, öS 1071,–
(Acta Neurochirurgica / Supplementum 36)
*Prices are subject to change without notice*

It has become increasingly difficult for single clinican to cover the whole area of traumatology and in particular neurotraumatology. This is now a science with many specialized fields of research and the results are published in many different journals, proceedings and books not easily available for those who are responsible for the daily practical management of patients with head injuries.
This volume considers all aspects, from accident and injury and their physical criteria, partly based on models and experimental animal designs, to epidemiology, pathophysiology, diagnosis, treatment and outcome. Particular attention is paid to the first general epidemiology study in specified populations as well as to data about longlasting residual disabilities gathered from insurance material. Classifications of head injuries in different systems are compared with regard to location, nature and severity and are discussed as a basis for ICD 10 (WHO). The defects in conscious reactions after head injuries are considered in clinical detail in various conscious reaction levels or "coma" scales and management charts are exemplified. New concepts with regard to serious posttraumatic longlasting defects of consciousness, particularly "vegetative" states, as well as for acute subdural hematoma of arterial origin are suggested. The different pictures of head injuries appearing in general hospital autopsy and forensic and clinical material are also discussed.
The volume will help to accumulate wider knowledge and better understanding between neurosurgeons and researchers in various neighboring fields to the benefit of the patients.

**Springer-Verlag Wien New York**
Moelkerbastei 5, A-1011 Wien
Heidelberger Platz 3, D-1000 Berlin 33
175 Fifth Avenue, New York, NY 10010 USA
37-3 Hongo 3-chome, Bunkyo-ku, Tokyo 113, Japan

GPSR Compliance

*The European Union's (EU) General Product Safety Regulation (GPSR) is a set of rules that requires consumer products to be safe and our obligations to ensure this.*

*If you have any concerns about our products, you can contact us on ProductSafety@springernature.com*

In case Publisher is established outside the EU, the EU authorized representative is:

Springer Nature Customer Service Center GmbH
Europaplatz 3
69115 Heidelberg, Germany

**Batch number: 10613743**

Printed by Printforce, the Netherlands